About the NCCN Guidelines for Patients®

NCCN National Comprehensive Cancer Network®

AF879051

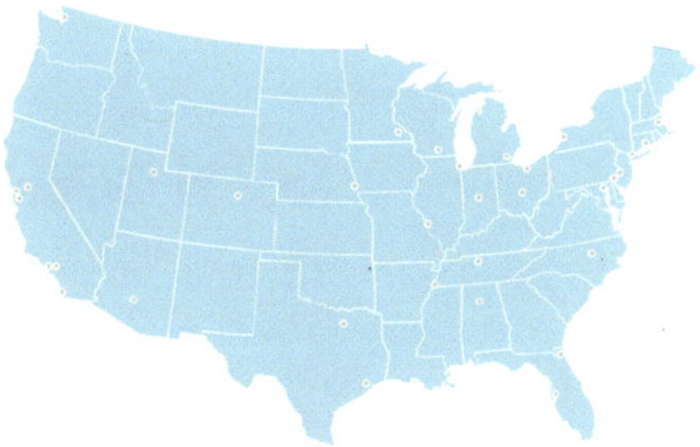

Did you know that top cancer centers across the United States work together to improve cancer care? This alliance of leading cancer centers is called the National Comprehensive Cancer Network® (NCCN®).

Cancer care is always changing. NCCN develops evidence-based cancer care recommendations used by health care providers worldwide. These frequently updated recommendations are the NCCN Clinical Practice Guidelines in Oncology (NCCN Guidelines®). The NCCN Guidelines for Patients plainly explain these expert recommendations for people with cancer and caregivers.

These NCCN Guidelines for Patients are based on the NCCN Clinical Practice Guidelines in Oncology (NCCN Guidelines®) for Hodgkin Lymphoma, Version 2.2023 – November 8, 2022.

View the NCCN Guidelines for Patients free online
NCCN.org/patientguidelines

Find an NCCN Cancer Center near you
NCCN.org/cancercenters

Connect with us YouTube

Supporters

NATIONAL COMPREHENSIVE CANCER NETWORK®
NCCN FOUNDATION
Guiding Treatment. Changing Lives.

NCCN Guidelines for Patients are supported by funding from the NCCN Foundation®

NCCN Foundation gratefully acknowledges the following corporate supporters for helping to make available these NCCN Guidelines for Patients: Bristol Myers Squibb and Seagen Inc.

NCCN independently adapts, updates, and hosts the NCCN Guidelines for Patients. Our corporate supporters do not participate in the development of the NCCN Guidelines for Patients and are not responsible for the content and recommendations contained therein.

To make a gift or learn more visit online or email

NCCNFoundation.org/donate

PatientGuidelines@NCCN.org

Contents

NCCN Foundation seeks to support the millions of patients and their families affected by a cancer diagnosis by funding and distributing NCCN Guidelines for Patients. NCCN Foundation is also committed to advancing cancer treatment by funding the nation's promising doctors at the center of innovation in cancer research. For more details and the full library of patient and caregiver resources, visit NCCN.org/patients.

National Comprehensive Cancer Network (NCCN) and NCCN Foundation
3025 Chemical Road, Suite 100, Plymouth Meeting, PA 19462 USA

1 Hodgkin lymphoma basics

Hodgkin lymphoma is an uncommon but highly curable cancer of the lymph nodes and the lymphatic system. More people survive Hodgkin lymphoma than any other cancer. Most people are diagnosed between the ages of 15 to 30, or after age 55.

The lymphatic system

The lymphatic system is a network of tissues and organs that help your body fight infection and disease. It is a major part of the body's immune system. The tissues and organs that make up the lymphatic system are made mostly of white blood cells called lymphocytes. There are four other types of white blood cells, but lymphocytes are the most important to understanding Hodgkin lymphoma.

Lymph and lymphatic vessels

There is a super-highway of ducts running through your body. These ducts are called lymphatic vessels. Much like how blood vessels transport blood, lymphatic vessels transport lymph. Lymph is a clear fluid that carries infection-fighting white blood cells (lymphocytes) throughout the body. It is also called lymphatic fluid.

Lymph nodes

While lymph travels throughout your body in lymphatic vessels, it passes through hundreds of small bean-shaped structures called lymph nodes. Lymph nodes catch and filter out foreign particles and harmful cells, including cancer cells. Lymph nodes can't usually be seen or felt. Certain areas of the body contain more lymph nodes than others. The highest numbers of lymph nodes are found in the:

- Neck (cervical lymph nodes)
- Groin (inguinal lymph nodes)
- Armpits (axillary lymph nodes)

Spleen

The spleen is the largest organ of the lymphatic system. It is about 4 inches long and shaped like a fist. It makes lymphocytes and plays an important role in blood filtration and storage.

Bone marrow

Most bones have soft, spongy tissue in the center called bone marrow. This is where new blood cells are made.

Thymus

After being made in bone marrow, lymphocytes travel to the thymus. The thymus is a small organ in the upper chest. Here lymphocytes develop into T lymphocytes (T cells), one of the two main types of lymphocytes.

The tonsils

Tonsils are small masses of lymph tissue found at the back of the throat. They help trap disease-causing germs that enter through your nose or mouth.

Lymphatic system

There are hundreds of small bean-shaped structures throughout the human body. They are called lymph nodes. Lymph nodes catch and filter out foreign particles and harmful cells, including cancer cells.

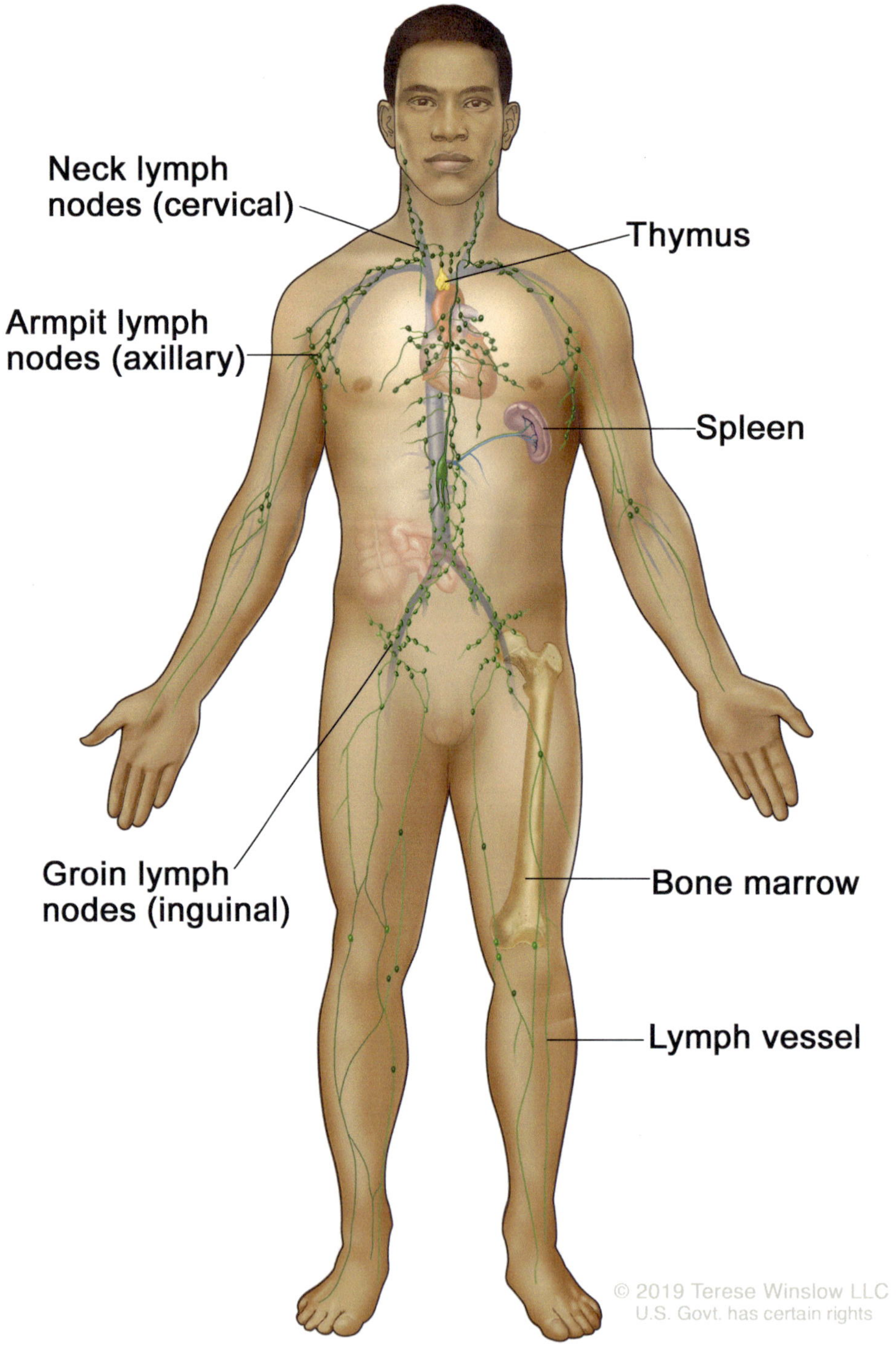

How Hodgkin lymphoma starts

The human body is made of trillions of cells. The cells grow, divide, and die as needed. Sometimes, however, errors occur when cells divide that causes them to start growing out of control. This is cancer. Lymphoma is cancer that begins when lymphocytes grow out of control.

Types of lymphoma

There are two main types of lymphoma:

- Non-Hodgkin lymphoma
- Hodgkin lymphoma

Doctors can tell if a suspected lymphoma is Hodgkin lymphoma by looking at one or more lymph nodes under a microscope. In Hodgkin lymphoma, the lymphocytes are abnormally large and may have more than one nucleus. These oversized lymphocytes are called Reed-Sternberg cells. Cancer researchers don't know why normal lymphocytes turn into Reed-Sternberg cells.

Non-Hodgkin lymphomas are a large and varied group of lymphomas. They do not have the distinctive Reed-Sternberg cells seen in Hodgkin lymphoma. **This book does not discuss treatment of non-Hodgkin lymphomas.**

Hodgkin lymphoma often spreads through lymphatic vessels from one group of lymph nodes to the next. If left untreated, it will spread to tissue and organs outside the lymphatic system.

Types of Hodgkin lymphoma

There are 2 types of Hodgkin lymphoma:

- Classic Hodgkin lymphoma (CHL)
- Nodular lymphocyte-predominant Hodgkin lymphoma (NLPHL)

CHL

Most people with Hodgkin lymphoma (about 95 out of 100) have CHL. CHL can be recognized by large lymphocytes called Reed-Sternberg cells.

There are 4 subtypes of CHL:

- Nodular sclerosis (most common)
- Mixed cellularity
- Lymphocyte-rich
- Lymphocyte-depleted (least common)

While they are all considered CHL, they look different under a microscope and have different features. For example, some are more likely to cause symptoms than others. The treatment information in this guide applies to all 4 subtypes. CHL is the focus of Part 4 beginning on page 31.

NLPHL

This type of Hodgkin lymphoma is rare. Only about 5 out of 100 people with Hodgkin lymphoma have NLPHL. While CHL is known for Reed-Sternberg cells, NLPHL is known for popcorn-shaped cells. NLPHL can be slow-growing in some patients, but in others it can behave aggressively. Over time, it can become a fast-growing type of non-Hodgkin lymphoma called diffuse large B-cell lymphoma (DLBCL). NLPHL is the focus of Part 5 beginning on page 40.

Key points

- CHL is a cancer of the lymph nodes and the lymphatic system. Most people with CHL are cured with chemotherapy.
- The lymphatic system is a network of vessels and organs made of white blood cells called lymphocytes. Lymphocytes help the body fight disease and infection.
- Cancer is the uncontrolled growth of cells. When lymphocytes grow out of control, the cancer is called a lymphoma.
- Hodgkin lymphoma starts in abnormally shaped lymphocytes called Reed-Sternberg cells.
- There are 2 types of Hodgkin lymphoma—CHL and NLPHL. CHL is the more common of the two.
- CHL has 4 subtypes: nodular sclerosis, mixed cellularity, lymphocyte-depleted, and lymphocyte-rich.
- The subtypes of CHL look different under a microscope and have different features.
- NLPHL is a rare form of Hodgkin lymphoma. It can transform into a fast-growing type of non-Hodgkin lymphoma.
- Hodgkin lymphoma often spreads from one group of lymph nodes to the next. If left untreated, it spreads to tissue and organs outside the lymphatic system.

We want your feedback!

Our goal is to provide helpful and easy-to-understand information on cancer.

Take our survey to let us know what we got right and what we could do better.

NCCN.org/patients/feedback

2

Testing for Hodgkin lymphoma

This chapter explains how Hodgkin lymphoma is identified (diagnosed). Other testing and care you may have before treatment is described.

Biopsy and lab testing

Excisional lymph node biopsy

The best way to diagnose Hodgkin lymphoma is to have one or more whole lymph nodes removed and tested. This is called an excisional lymph node biopsy. This method is the most accurate because it allows entire lymph nodes to be tested, not just samples taken from inside the lymph nodes.

Needle biopsies

While an excisional lymph node biopsy is preferred, another type of biopsy called a core needle biopsy may be done in some cases. In a core needle biopsy, a surgeon uses a wide needle to remove a sample of tissue from a lymph node, but does not remove the entire lymph node.

A third type of biopsy called a fine-needle aspiration (FNA) should not be used alone to diagnose Hodgkin lymphoma. In an FNA biopsy, a thin needle is used to remove a sample of tissue from a lymph node, but does not remove the entire lymph node. While widely used to diagnose other types of cancer, it is not used by itself to diagnose Hodgkin lymphoma.

Testing the removed lymph node(s)

The removed lymph nodes are tested using a process called immunohistochemistry (IHC). Using a microscope, this test looks for proteins on the surface of cells. A diagnosis can be made based on the proteins that can be seen (and not seen) using this technique. For example, if you have CHL, proteins called CD15 and CD30 can usually be seen during immunohistochemistry, but CD3 and CD45 usually cannot.

Health history and physical exam

Expect your doctor to review your health history and perform a complete physical exam. These are important first steps in planning your cancer treatment.

Symptoms

Hodgkin lymphoma can cause symptoms. There are three symptoms in particular that are important for your doctor to be aware of, if you have them. These are called B symptoms or systemic symptoms.

The B symptoms are:

- Unexplained high fevers (above 100.4 degrees Fahrenheit)
- Heavy, drenching night sweats
- Loss of more than 10 percent of your body weight without dieting

There are other symptoms that may be related to Hodgkin lymphoma. Tell your doctor if you have any of the symptoms listed below.

- Itchy skin (pruritus)
- Extreme tiredness despite sleep (fatigue)
- A bad reaction to alcohol

Physical exam

While lymph nodes can't usually be seen or felt, Hodgkin lymphoma can cause them to get bigger. Using their hands, your doctor will feel the areas of your body where there are the most lymph nodes. This includes the neck, armpits, and groin. In addition to examining areas where there are many lymph nodes, expect your doctor to feel your spleen and liver.

Performance status

Your doctor will also rate your performance status. This is your ability to do daily tasks and activities. It is used by doctors to decide if you can have certain treatments.

Hodgkin lymphoma B symptoms

Fever

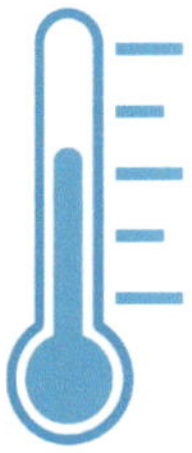

Heavy night sweats

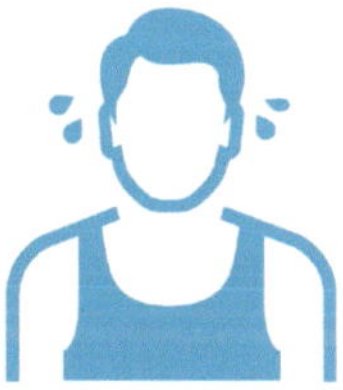

Unexplained weight loss

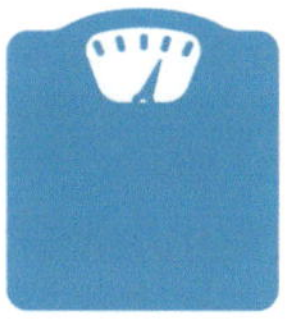

Blood tests

Blood tests are included in the workup (testing) for Hodgkin lymphoma. These common tests are described next.

- **Complete blood count (CBC).** This test measures the number of red blood cells, white blood cells, and platelets in a sample of blood.
- **Erythrocyte sedimentation rate (ESR).** This test measures how quickly red blood cells settle at the bottom of a test tube that contains a blood sample. A faster-than-normal ESR may be a sign of inflammation, infection, cancer, or other diseases.
- **Comprehensive metabolic panel (CMP).** This group of more than 10 blood tests provides information about the health of your kidneys, bones, and other organs and tissues. It also gives information on your blood sugar, calcium, and electrolytes.
- **Liver function tests.** These tests are often done along with a CMP. The liver is an organ that does many important jobs, such as remove toxins from the blood. Liver function tests measure enzymes that are made or processed by the liver.
- **Serum lactate dehydrogenase (LDH).** A high level of this protein in blood can be a sign of cell damage caused by cancer or other health problems.

Your doctor may also suggest testing your blood for human immunodeficiency virus (HIV) and for hepatitis B or C. This is encouraged, especially if your doctor thinks you may be at risk for these diseases.

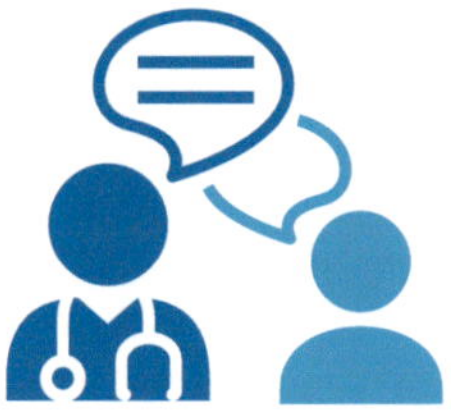

Receiving your test results

Think about how you want to receive your test results. Share your thoughts with your care team. Accessing results online using a patient portal is often an option. But, understanding testing reports can be confusing and may even be stressful. You may prefer for your doctor to convey results in person or over the phone. Let your care team how you would like to receive information.

Imaging tests

PET/CT scan

A positron emission tomography/computed tomography (PET/CT) scan combines the use of two tests (PET and CT). Some cancer centers have one machine that does both. This is called an integrated PET/CT. Often, however, the CT part of an integrated PET/CT is not done with contrast. Contrast is a substance that makes the pictures clearer. In some cases a separate CT with contrast may also be needed.

PET scans use a small amount of radioactive glucose (sugar), called a radiotracer. Fluorodeoxyglucose (FDG) is the most commonly used radiotracer. The radiotracer gives off a small amount of energy that is detected by the PET/CT machine. Areas with cancer appear brighter ("hotter") because cancer cells use sugar more quickly than normal cells. However, these "hot spots" can be caused by health conditions other than cancer.

CT takes many pictures of a body part from different angles using x-rays. A computer combines the x-rays to make detailed pictures. The contrast will be injected into your vein. You will be asked a series of questions to make sure you are not allergic to the contrast. Allergic reactions include throat swelling and hives. CT of your neck is needed if your neck may be treated with radiation. Any areas that look abnormal on PET/CT should also be imaged.

PET scans play a key role in the management of Hodgkin lymphoma. It is common to have more than one PET scan during the course of treatment. They are used to determine the stage of disease and to see how well treatment is working. Keep in mind that PET scans may be abnormal if you have an infection, inflammation, or other conditions, even if you don't have Hodgkin lymphoma.

PET/CT

PET scans play a key role in the management of Hodgkin lymphoma. They are used to determine the stage of disease and to see how well treatment is working.

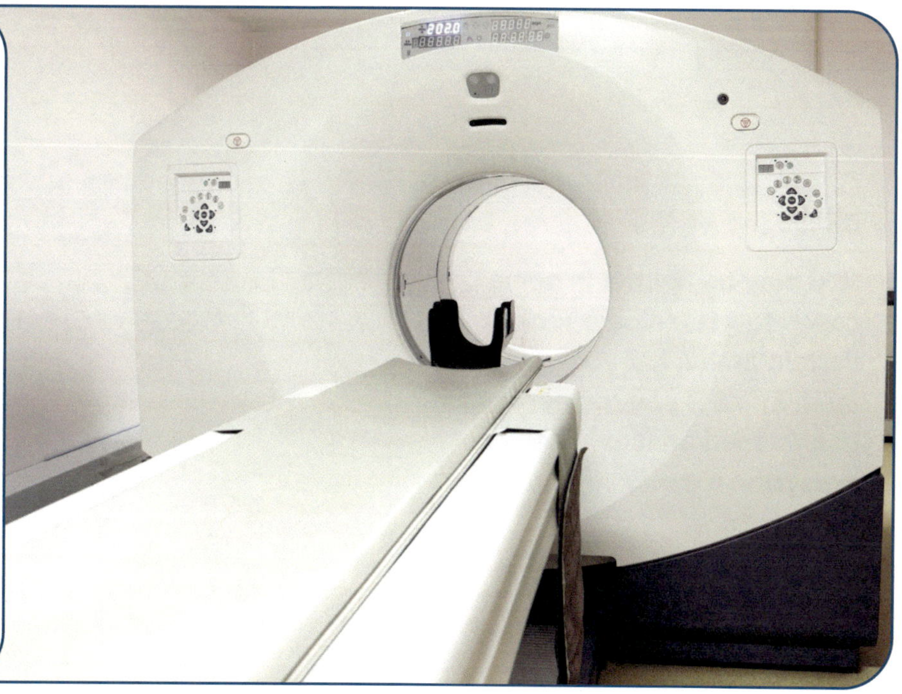

Deauville scores

A scoring system is used to describe how much of the tracer is absorbed by areas with cancer compared to how much is absorbed by your liver and by the area between the lungs (but not the lungs themselves). This area is called the mediastinum. There are 5 possible scores (called Deauville scores), ranging from 1 to 5. A score of 1 or 2 is generally considered "negative." This means that there are no cancerous areas of concern. A score of 4 or 5 is generally considered "positive." This means that there are cancerous areas of concern. A score of 3 can be considered positive or negative, depending on the situation.

The Deauville score given when you are first diagnosed is not important. **Whether that score goes up or down as a result of treatment is important.** This is how doctors know how well treatment is working.

Other imaging

A chest x-ray can help spot enlarged lymph nodes in the chest. It may be the first diagnostic test performed. The findings of a chest x-ray typically need to be confirmed with further imaging.

Magnetic resonance imaging (MRI) may be helpful in some cases to get a closer look at certain areas. It may also be used in combination with PET (a PET/MRI). Let your care team know if you are afraid of enclosed spaces. There are medications that can help.

MRI

MRI may be helpful in some cases to get a closer look at certain areas. Let your care team know if you get nervous in enclosed spaces. They can prescribe a medication that can help.

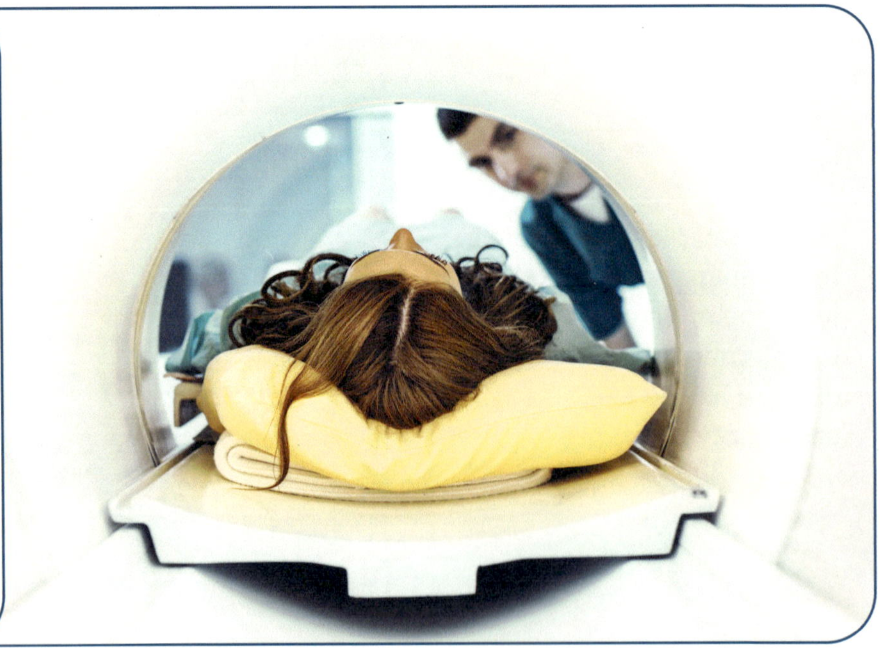

Heart and lung tests

Some cancer treatments can damage your heart and lungs. In order to plan your treatment, your doctors will test how well your heart and lungs work.

Ejection fraction

An echocardiogram is an imaging test of your heart. It can provide important information, including how much blood is pumped out of the left side of your heart every time it beats. This is called the ejection fraction. A high or low ejection fraction may mean you can't have certain chemotherapy medicines.

Lung function tests

Bleomycin (Blenoxane) is a chemotherapy medicine often used to treat Hodgkin lymphoma. Bleomycin can damage the lungs and cause a disease called pulmonary fibrosis. In order to learn if your lungs can handle treatment with bleomycin, you should have lung testing before starting treatment. The three most common lung function tests are described below.

- **Spirometry** measures the amount of air the lungs can hold, and how fast you can empty the air out of your lungs.
- **A gas diffusion test** involves breathing in a harmless gas and measuring how much of it you breathe out. It tells how much oxygen travels from your lungs into your blood.
- **Body plethysmograph** involves sitting in a small room and breathing into a tube. This test measures how much air your lungs can hold and how much air is left in your lungs after you exhale.

Echocardiogram

An echocardiogram is one way of measuring ejection fraction, which is the amount of blood pumped out of the left side of your heart each time it beats. Measurement of ejection fraction is recommended for most people before starting anthracycline-based chemotherapy.

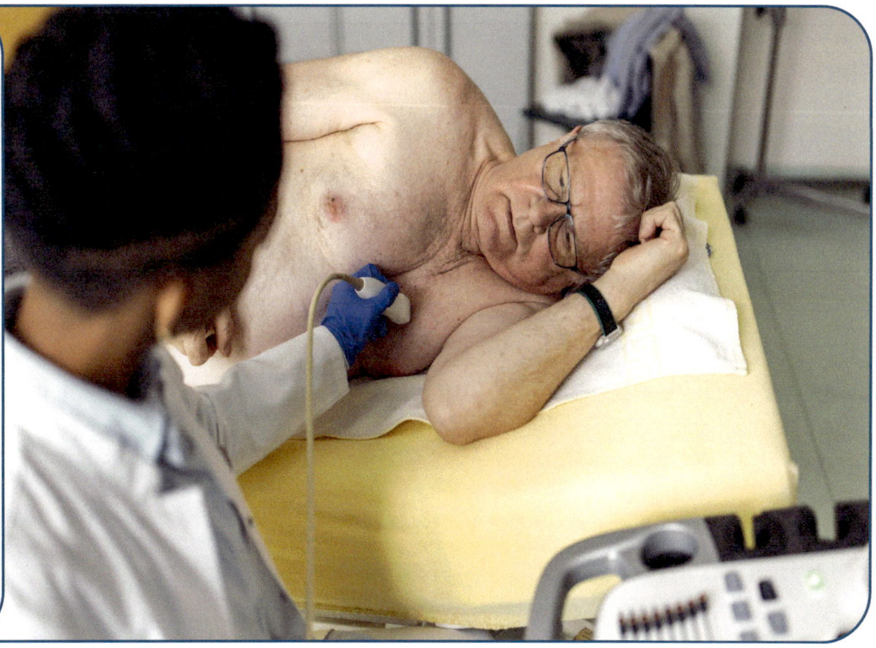

Other testing and care

Help to quit smoking

If you smoke, it is important to quit. Smoking can limit how well cancer treatment works. Smoking and vaping can also increase the risk of lung problems during chemotherapy. If you smoke, ask your doctor about counseling and drugs to help you quit.

Fertility and pregnancy

Some chemotherapy regimens (eg, BEACOPP) can cause immediate and permanent infertility. Other chemotherapy regimens (eg, ABVD) rarely cause infertility. Most people will have chemotherapy with a regimen that is unlikely to cause infertility.

If you want the option of having children after treatment or are unsure, tell your doctors. There are ways to be able to have children after treatment. This is called fertility preservation. The most common methods of fertility preservation are described next. In addition, anyone diagnosed with Hodgkin lymphoma who could become pregnant should expect to be tested for pregnancy before starting treatment.

Sperm banking

Sperm banking stores semen for later use by freezing it in liquid nitrogen. The medical term for this is semen cryopreservation.

Egg freezing

Like sperm banking, unfertilized eggs can be removed, frozen, and stored for later use. The medical term for this is oocyte cryopreservation.

Ovarian tissue banking

This method involves removing part or all of an ovary and freezing the part that contains the eggs. The frozen tissue that contains the eggs can later be unfrozen and put back in the body.

More information on fertility preservation in adolescents and young adults is available at NCCN.org/patientguidelines and on the NCCN Patient Guides for Cancer app.

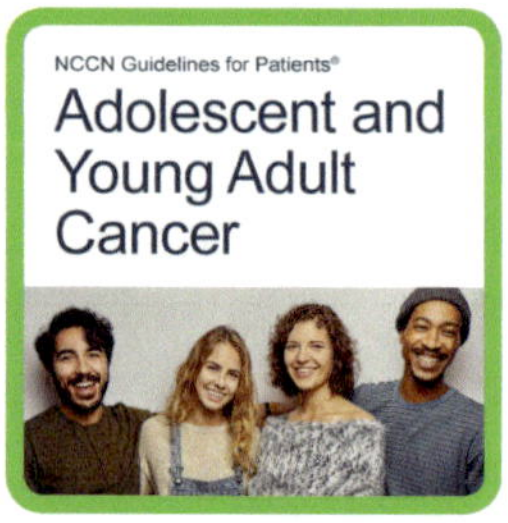

Vaccines

Everyone should get the influenza vaccine (the "flu shot") and other vaccines as needed. This includes the COVID-19 vaccine. NCCN offers more information on COVID-19 at NCCN.org/covid-19.

Your spleen is part of your lymphatic system. If your spleen is treated with radiation, your chances of getting an infection are increased. In this case, get vaccinated before treatment against pneumonia, meningitis, and Haemophilus influenzae type B ("Hib" or "H-flu"). Despite its name, the H-flu does not cause the common flu. It most often causes pneumonia, but can cause many different kinds of infections.

Bone marrow biopsy

In general, bone marrow biopsies are no longer included in the initial testing for Hodgkin lymphoma. However, if you have lower-than-normal numbers of blood cells and a PET scan doesn't suggest there is cancer in the marrow, a bone marrow biopsy may be needed.

The power of support

Seek out support groups at your treatment center, through social media, or from the resources listed in the back of this book. Look to friends, relatives, neighbors, and co-workers for social support. Many people find support groups helpful even after treatment is over. It can help with anxiety about cancer returning (recurrence).

Support is available for those affected by cancer that may have unique needs, including:

- Adolescents and young adults ("AYAs") with cancer
- Families and friends of people living with cancer

Staging

Before starting treatment, it is important to know how far the cancer has spread. This process is called staging. The testing described earlier in this chapter is used to determine the stage (extent) of the cancer.

Hodgkin lymphoma usually starts in the upper body–often in lymph nodes in the neck, chest, or armpits. The diaphragm is a thin muscle below the lungs and heart. It can be thought of as a dividing line between the chest and the abdomen. **Hodgkin lymphoma is staged in part depending on whether cancer has spread to lymph nodes or other areas below the diaphragm.**

There are 4 stages of Hodgkin lymphoma (I, II, III, and IV). A simplified description of the stages is provided next. The stages are described in more detail on the next pages.

If there is cancer in only one group of lymph nodes, the cancer is stage I. If the cancer spreads to more lymph but stays on the same side of the diaphragm, it is stage II. If Hodgkin lymphoma spreads to lymph nodes above and below the diaphragm, it is stage III. Hodgkin lymphoma that has spread to one or more areas outside of the lymphatic system is stage IV.

For the purposes of treatment, the stages are often grouped together as follows after diagnosis and initial workup:

- Stage I–II
- Stage III–IV

An "A" after the stage means that there aren't B symptoms. A "B" after the stage means that there are B symptoms. Unexplained fevers, drenching night sweats, and extreme weight loss are B symptoms.

Stage I

There is cancer in one group of lymph nodes, and possibly in one small area or organ outside the lymphatic system.

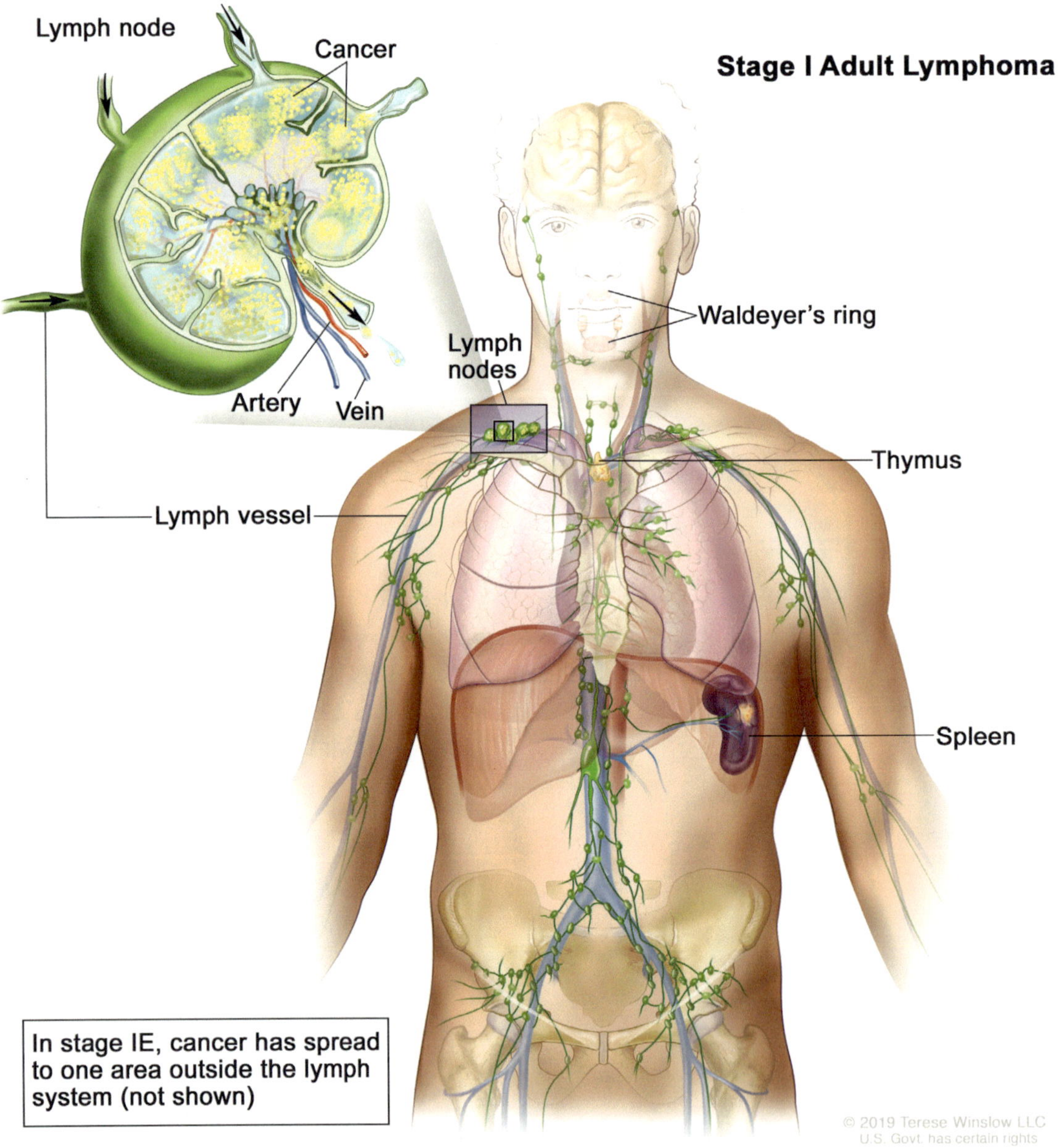

Stage II

There is cancer in 2 or more groups of lymph nodes on the same side (above or below) of the diaphragm, and possibly in one area or organ and its nearby lymph nodes outside the lymphatic system.

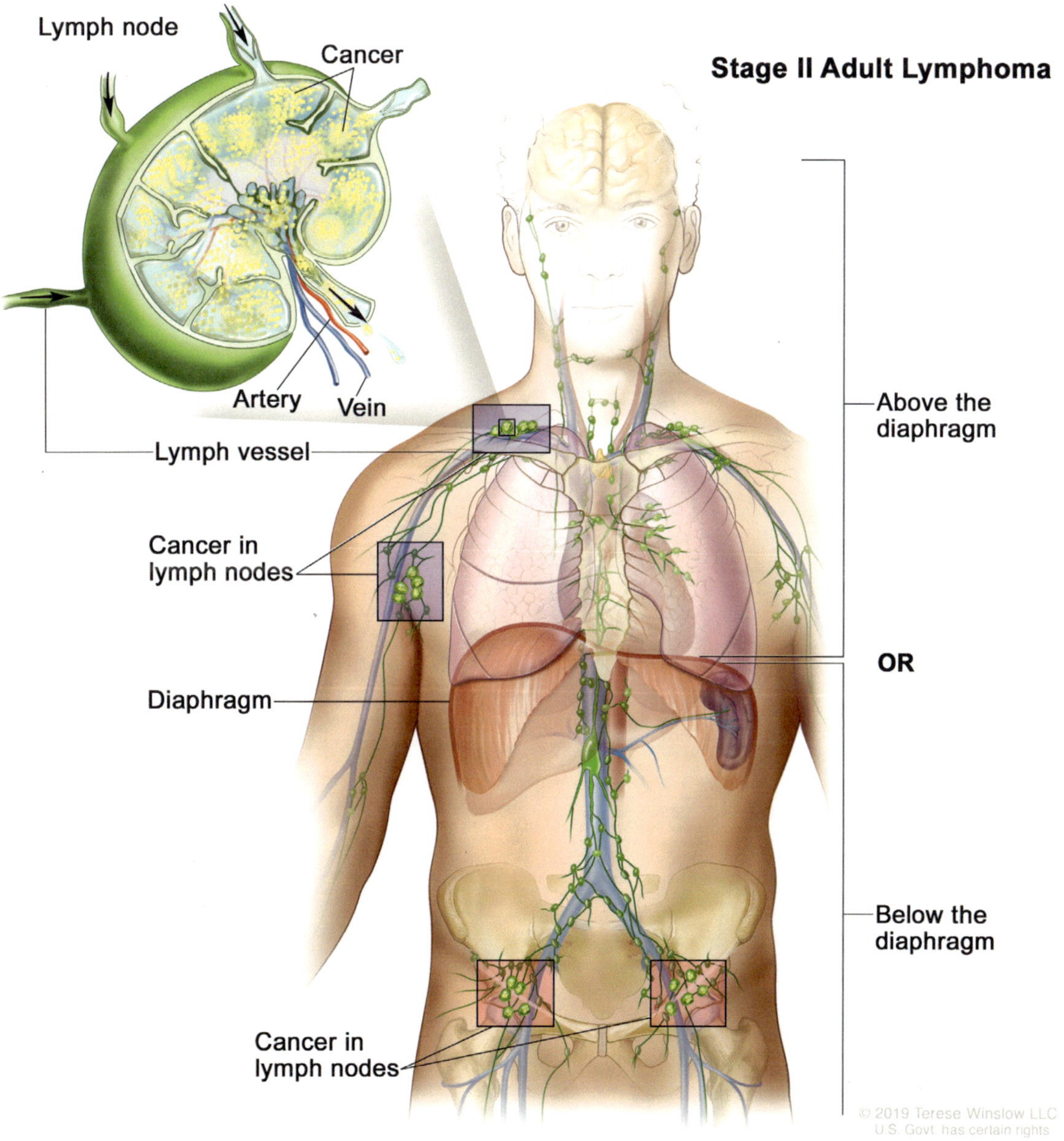

Stage III

There is cancer in lymph nodes on both sides (above and below) of the diaphragm. There may also be cancer in one area or organ outside of the lymphatic system, in the spleen, or both.

Stage III Adult Lymphoma

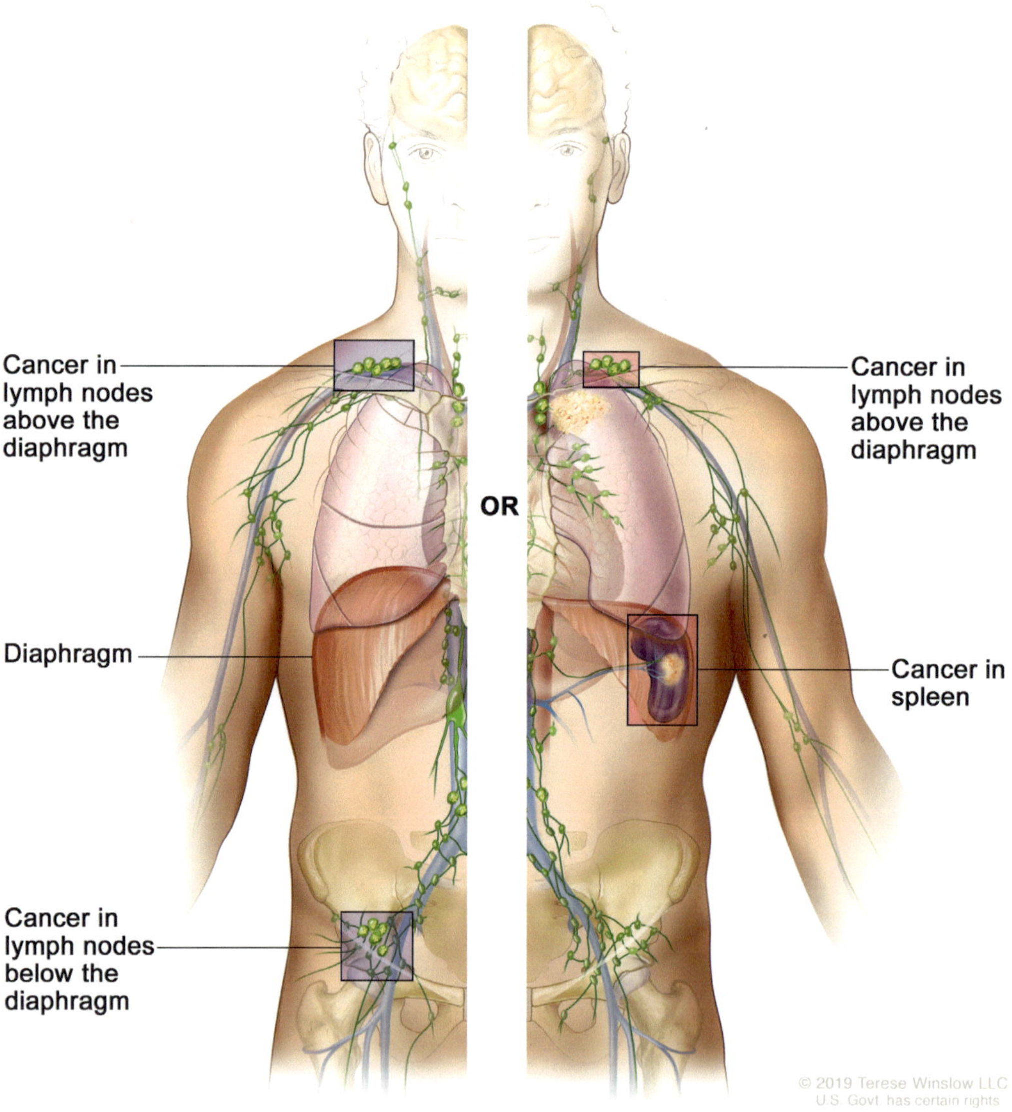

Stage IV

There are multiple areas of cancer in one or more organs outside the lymphatic system, and possibly in the neighboring lymph nodes. Or, there may be cancer in one organ outside of the lymphatic system and also in distant lymph nodes.

Stage IV Adult Lymphoma

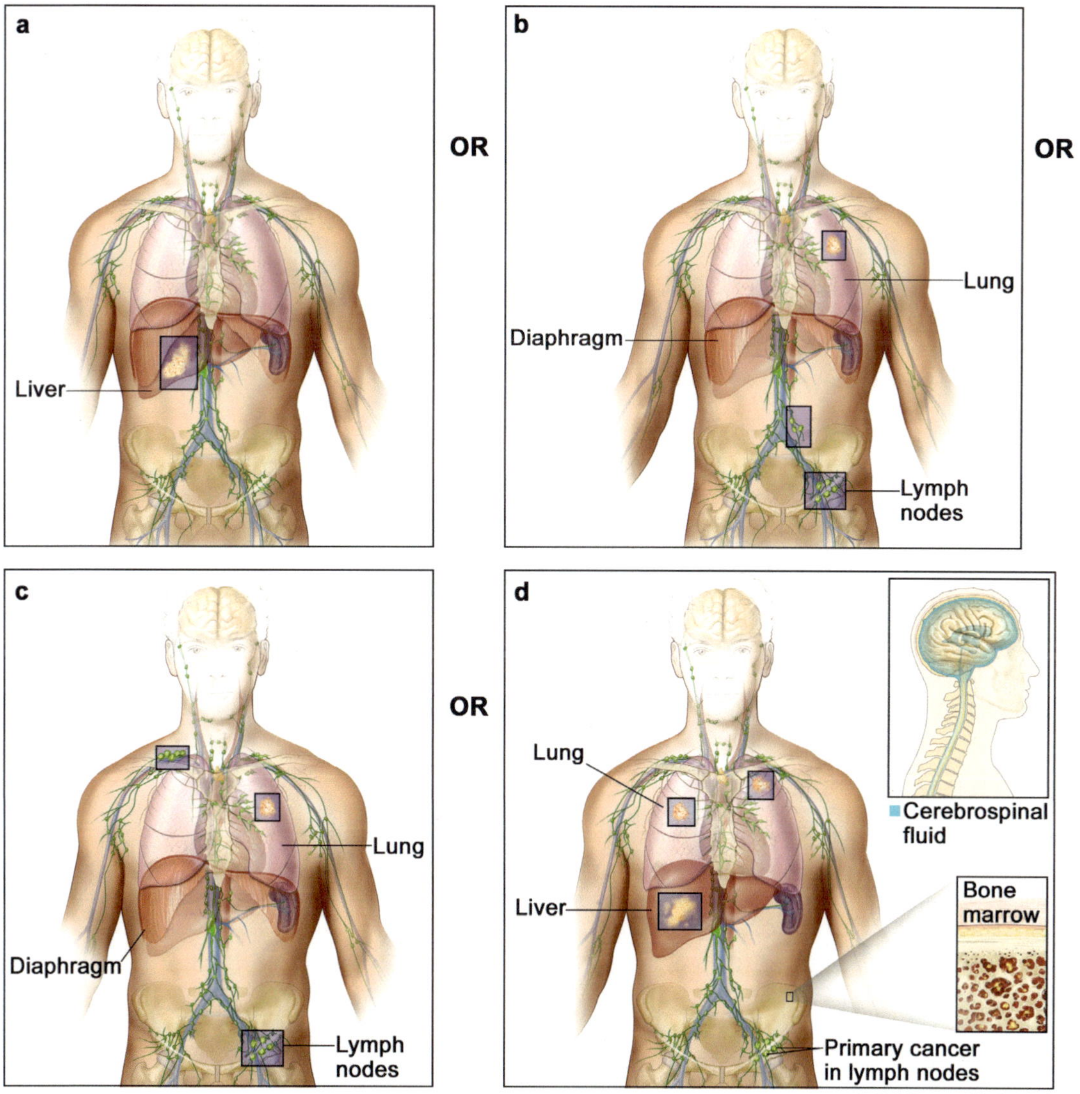

Key points

- An excisional lymph node biopsy is the most accurate way to diagnose Hodgkin lymphoma.
- Hodgkin lymphoma can cause unexplained high fevers, drenching night sweats, and extreme weight loss without dieting. These are called B symptoms.
- Other possible symptoms include itchy skin, extreme tiredness, and having a bad reaction to alcohol.
- Blood tests for Hodgkin lymphoma include a CBC, ESR, comprehensive metabolic panel, liver function tests, and measurement of lactate dehydrogenase.
- PET/CT scans are used to determine the stage of disease and to see how well Hodgkin lymphoma is responding to treatment.
- Most people with Hodgkin lymphoma need testing of their heart and lungs. This helps determine if they can have certain chemotherapy medicines.
- Most people are treated with chemotherapy that is unlikely to cause infertility. However, fertility preservation methods are available if a regimen that may impair fertility is planned.
- You may need to receive vaccinations to protect you from illness during cancer treatment.
- If you smoke, ask your doctor for help to quit.
- There are 4 stages of Hodgkin lymphoma (I, II, III, and IV).
- In stage I, there is cancer in one group of lymph nodes. There may also be cancer in one small area or organ outside the lymphatic system.
- In stage II, there is cancer in 2 or more groups of lymph nodes on the same side of the diaphragm (either above or below). There may also be cancer in one area or organ and its nearby lymph nodes outside the lymphatic system.
- In stage III, there is cancer in lymph nodes on both sides of the diaphragm. There may also be cancer in one area or organ outside of the lymphatic system, in the spleen, or both.
- In stage IV, there are multiple areas of cancer in organs outside the lymphatic system, and possibly in the neighboring lymph nodes.

3

Treatments for Hodgkin lymphoma

This chapter briefly describes the cancer treatments used for Hodgkin lymphoma. Chemotherapy is the most widely used and most effective treatment for this cancer.

Systemic therapy

Systemic therapy is the use of medicine to kill cancer cells. It is the most widely used treatment for Hodgkin lymphoma. Chemotherapy, targeted therapy, and immunotherapy are types of systemic therapy.

Most systemic therapies are liquids that are slowly injected into a vein. This process is called infusion. The drugs travel in your bloodstream to treat cancer throughout the body. Systemic therapy also harms healthy cells, which is why it can cause harsh side effects.

Systemic therapy is given in cycles of treatment days followed by days of rest. This allows the body to recover before the next cycle. Cycles vary in length depending on which drugs are used. Systemic therapies may be given alone or combined.

Chemotherapy

Classic Hodgkin lymphoma (CHL) is usually treated with chemotherapy. Other types of systemic therapy may be given with chemotherapy. Commonly used regimens are listed in **Guide 1.**

Some chemotherapy regimens include steroids. Steroids are drugs that relieve inflammation, but that also have anti-cancer effects. Steroids used with chemotherapy to treat Hodgkin lymphoma include dexamethasone and prednisone.

Guide 1
Commonly used chemotherapy regimens for CHL

ABVD	Doxorubicin (Adriamycin), bleomycin (Blenoxane), vinblastine, and dacarbazine
AVD	Doxorubicin, vinblastine, and dacarbazine
BV + AVD	Brentuximab vedotin (Adcetris) + AVD
Escalated BEACOPP	Bleomycin, etoposide (Etopophos), doxorubicin, cyclophosphamide, vincristine, procarbazine (Matulane), and prednisone

Brentuximab vedotin (Adcetris)

Brentuximab is an antibody drug conjugate. This means it combines two drugs in one medicine. The antibody component (brentuximab) finds and attaches to cancer cells that have a specific protein (CD30) on their surface. Once attached, a chemotherapy drug is released into the cancer cell. By targeting only cells with CD30 receptors, fewer normal cells are harmed.

Brentuximab vedotin is a treatment option for CHL that does not respond to treatment (refractory) or that returns after treatment (relapsed). It is also an option for first-line treatment of advanced (stage III-IV) CHL in combination with chemotherapy. It is put directly into the bloodstream (infusion).

Immunotherapy

Your immune system is your body's natural defense against infection and disease. Immunotherapy is a cancer treatment that increases the activity of your immune system. By doing so, it improves the body's ability to find and destroy cancer cells. Immunotherapy medicines called checkpoint inhibitors may be used to treat refractory or relapsed Hodgkin lymphoma. They include nivolumab (Opdivo) and pembrolizumab (Keytruda). More information on the side effects of checkpoint inhibitors is available at NCCN.org/patientguidelines and on the NCCN Patient Guides for Cancer app.

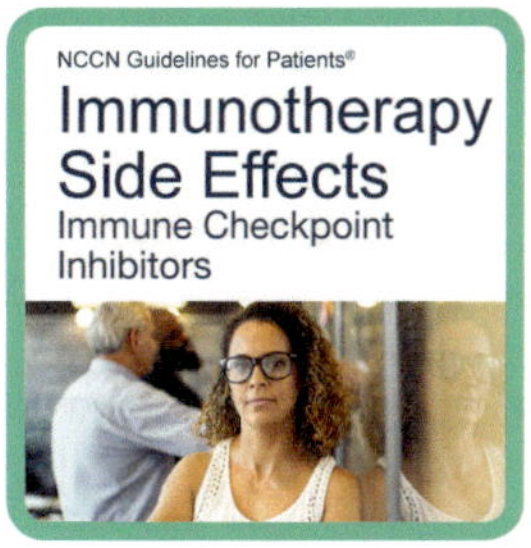

Rituximab (Rituxan)

Rituximab is an antibody therapy used to treat nodular lymphocyte-predominant Hodgkin lymphoma (NLPHL). NLPHL cells (and some healthy blood cells) have a protein on their surface called CD20. Rituximab targets and attaches to the CD20 protein. This helps your immune system find and attack the cancer cells. Rituximab may be given alone or with chemotherapy to treat NLPHL.

Side effects

Managing side effects is a shared effort between you and your care team. It is important to speak up about bothersome side effects, such as nausea and vomiting. Ask about your options for managing or relieving the effects of treatment.

More information on nausea and vomiting is available at NCCN.org/patientguidelines and on the NCCN Patient Guides for Cancer app.

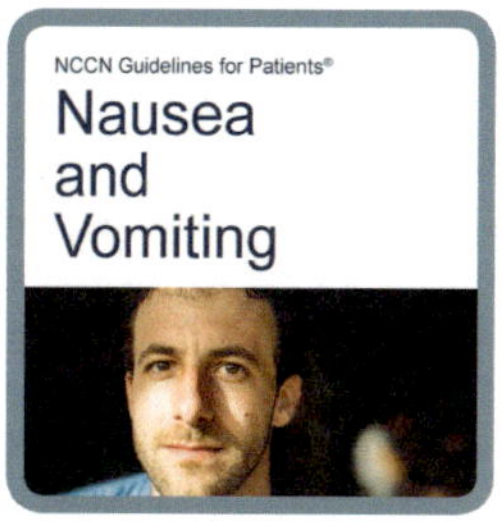

Radiation therapy

Radiation therapy is often used in addition to chemotherapy to treat Hodgkin lymphoma. It is also sometimes used alone. Using high-energy x-rays (photons), radiation therapy kills existing cancer cells or stops new cancer cells from being made. Radiation can also harm normal cells.

In some cases, particle-based radiation therapy (such as proton therapy) may be used. This is especially true for younger people with lymphoma in the area of the chest between the lungs (the mediastinum). Proton therapy may reduce late side effects caused by treatment with radiation. Such late effects include heart disease and second cancers.

Involved-site radiation therapy (ISRT)

Involved-site radiation therapy (ISRT) is recommended to treat Hodgkin lymphoma. ISRT targets the lymph nodes in which the cancer first started and nearby areas of cancer. ISRT is a type of external beam radiation therapy (EBRT). External radiation simply means that the radiation comes from a machine outside of (external to) your body.

A simulation session is required if radiation therapy is planned. It is performed before the start of radiation therapy. During simulation, pictures of the tumor will be taken. This is usually done using a CT scan in the radiation treatment position. The pictures are used to plan the best radiation dose, number and shape of radiation beams, and number of treatment sessions. You may be asked to hold your breath during the simulation scan or treatment in order to limit the movement of your heart and lungs. During treatment, you will lie on a table in the same position as done

Radiation therapy

Radiation therapy is usually used in addition to chemotherapy to treat Hodgkin lymphoma. A type of external radiation therapy called involved-site radiation therapy (ISRT) targets the lymph nodes where the cancer started and nearby areas of cancer.

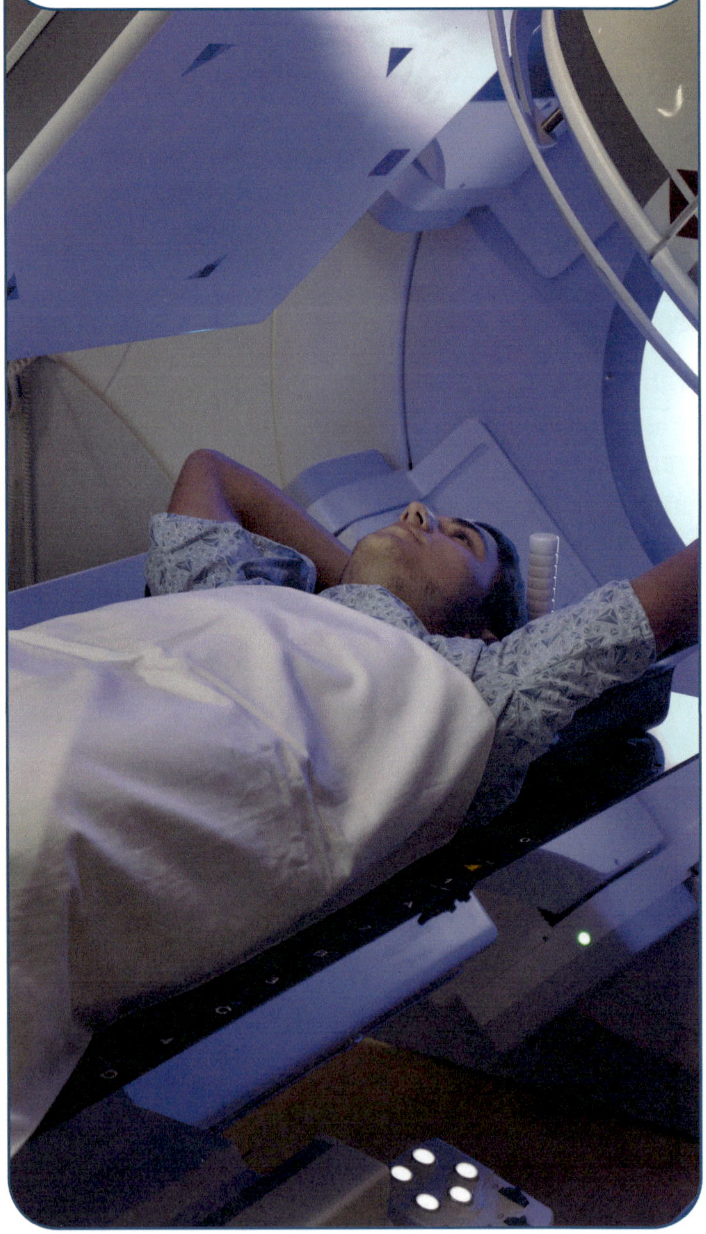

for simulation. Devices may be used to keep you from moving. These may include a mesh mask and body mold. You will be alone while the therapists operate the machine from a nearby control room.

If treatment with radiation therapy is planned, adolescents and young adults are encouraged to ask if proton therapy is right for them.

High-dose chemotherapy with stem cell rescue

Red blood cells, white blood cells, and platelets are the three main types of blood cells. Each has a different and important job in the body. Red blood cells carry oxygen. White blood cells fight infection. Platelets help stop bleeding.

Before becoming one of these types, all blood cells start as "stem" cells. Stem cells that become blood cells are known as hematopoietic stem cells. Hematopoietic (blood-forming) stem cells are found in bone marrow. When hematopoietic stem cells are damaged, they may not form the blood cells needed by the body.

Autologous stem cell transplant

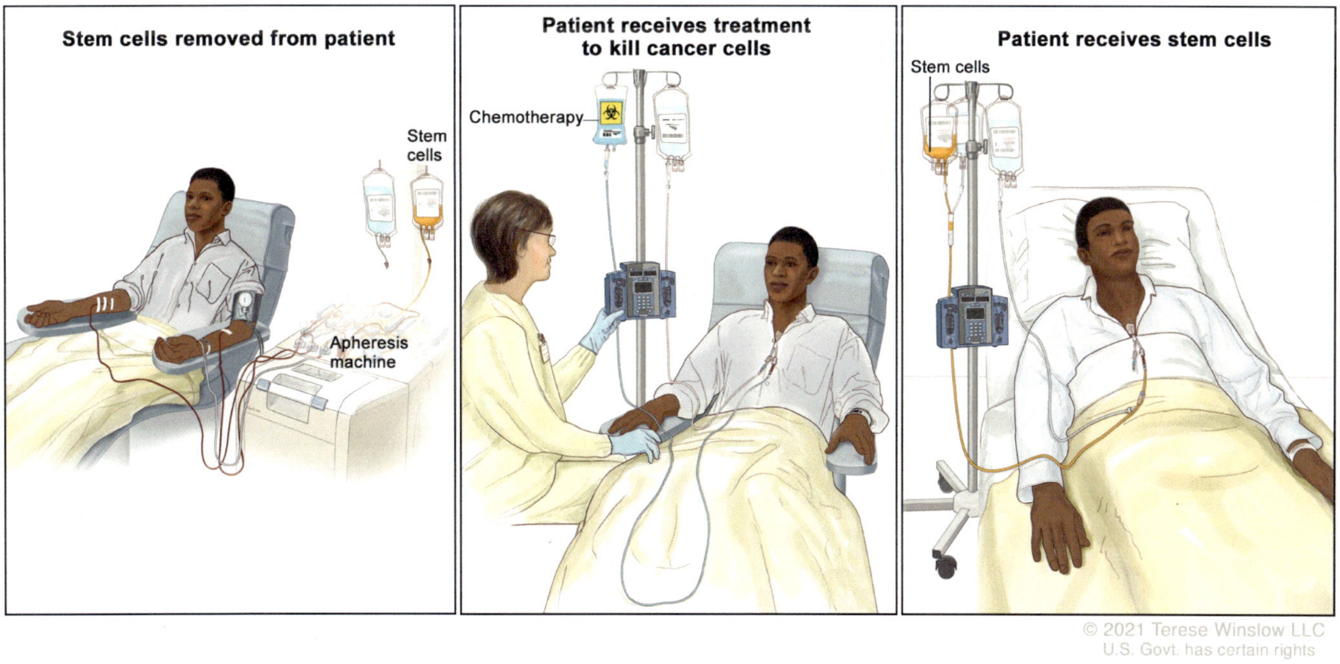

High-dose chemotherapy can damage or destroy hematopoietic stem cells. High-dose chemotherapy may be used for Hodgkin lymphoma that does not respond to treatment. To protect your blood-forming stem cells from high-dose chemotherapy, they are first removed ("rescued") from your blood or bone marrow.

After chemotherapy, your rescued, healthy stem cells are transplanted back into your body. The transplanted stem cells form new red blood cells, white blood cells, and platelets. This restores your body's ability to protect itself from infection.

A number of names are used to refer to this procedure, including:

- Autologous bone marrow transplant
- Autologous stem cell transplant
- Hematopoietic cell transplant (HCT)
- High-dose therapy with autologous stem cell rescue (HDT/ASCR)

The stem cell rescue process

The first step is to increase the number of stem cells in the blood. This is known as "mobilization." Medicines are used to cause stem cells to move from the bone marrow into the blood. When your doctor determines that your stem cell count is high enough, the next step is collection.

A process called apheresis is used to collect the stem cells from blood. Your blood will be removed from a large vein, most likely in your arm. It will flow through a tube and into a machine that removes stem cells. The rest of your blood will be returned to you in your other arm. Apheresis typically takes 4 to 6 hours and does not require anesthesia. It may take two or more sessions to obtain enough stem cells. During the procedure, you may have lightheadedness, chills, numbness around the lips, and cramping in the hands. After apheresis, the collected ("harvested") cells are frozen and stored.

When high-dose chemotherapy is complete, your harvested stem cells will be put back into your body using a transfusion. A transfusion is a slow injection of blood products through a central line into a large vein. A central line (or central venous catheter) is a thin tube. The tube will be inserted into your skin through one incision (cut), then into your vein through a second cut. Local anesthesia will be used. This process can take several hours to complete.

The transplanted stem cells travel to your bone marrow where they grow and form new, healthy blood cells. This is called engraftment. It usually takes about 2 to 4 weeks. Until engraftment is fully achieved, you will have little or no immune defense. You will need to stay in a very clean room at the hospital. You may be given an antibiotic to prevent or treat infection. You may also be given blood transfusions to prevent bleeding and to treat low red blood counts (anemia) and low platelets (thrombocytopenia). While waiting for the cells to engraft, you will likely feel tired and weak.

Allogeneic stem cell transplant

An allogeneic stem cell transplant uses stem cells from a donor. This type of stem cell transplant is not used often for CHL, but may be an option for CHL that doesn't respond to treatment.

Clinical trials

A clinical trial is a type of medical research study. After being developed and tested in a laboratory, potential new ways of fighting cancer need to be studied in people. If found to be safe and effective in a clinical trial, a drug, device, or treatment approach may be approved by the U.S. Food and Drug Administration (FDA).

Everyone with cancer should carefully consider all of the treatment options available for their cancer type, including standard treatments and clinical trials. Talk to your doctor about whether a clinical trial may make sense for you.

Phases

Most cancer clinical trials focus on treatment. Treatment trials are done in phases.

- **Phase I trials** study the dose, safety, and side effects of an investigational drug or treatment approach. They also look for early signs that the drug or approach is helpful.
- **Phase II trials** study how well the drug or approach works against a specific type of cancer.
- **Phase III trials** test the drug or approach against a standard treatment. If the results are good, it may be approved by the FDA.
- **Phase IV trials** study the long-term safety and benefit of an FDA-approved treatment.

Who can enroll?

Every clinical trial has rules for joining, called eligibility criteria. The rules may be about age, cancer type and stage, treatment history, or general health. These requirements ensure that participants are alike in specific ways and that the trial is as safe as possible for the participants.

Finding a clinical trial

In the United States

NCCN Cancer Centers
NCCN.org/cancercenters

The National Cancer Institute (NCI)
cancer.gov/about-cancer/treatment/clinical-trials/search

Worldwide

The U.S. National Library of Medicine (NLM)
clinicaltrials.gov/

Need help finding a clinical trial?

NCI's Cancer Information Service (CIS)
1.800.4.CANCER (1.800.422.6237)
cancer.gov/contact

Informed consent

Clinical trials are managed by a group of experts called a research team. The research team will review the study with you in detail, including its purpose and the risks and benefits of joining. All of this information is also provided in an informed consent form. Read the form carefully and ask questions before signing it. Take time to discuss it with family, friends, or others you trust. Keep in mind that you can leave and seek treatment outside of the clinical trial at any time.

Start the conversation

Don't wait for your doctor to bring up clinical trials. Start the conversation and learn about all of your treatment options. If you find a study that you may be eligible for, ask your treatment team if you meet the requirements. If you have already started standard treatment, you may not be eligible for certain clinical trials. Try not to be discouraged if you cannot join. New clinical trials are always becoming available.

Frequently asked questions

There are many myths and misconceptions surrounding clinical trials. The possible benefits and risks are not well understood by many with cancer.

Will I get a placebo?

Placebos (inactive versions of real medicines) are almost never used alone in cancer clinical trials. It is common to receive either a placebo with a standard treatment or a new drug with a standard treatment. You will be informed, verbally and in writing, if a placebo is part of a clinical trial before you enroll.

Are clinical trials free?

There is no fee to enroll in a clinical trial. The study sponsor pays for research-related costs, including the study drug. You may, however, have costs indirectly related to the trial, such as the cost of transportation or child care due to extra appointments. During the trial, you will continue to receive standard cancer care. This care is billed to—and often covered by—insurance. You are responsible for copays and any costs for this care that are not covered by your insurance.

Key points

- Chemotherapy is the most widely used and most effective treatment for Hodgkin lymphoma.
- Some steroids have anti-cancer effects and may be used with chemotherapy.
- Radiation therapy is often given after chemotherapy but sometimes is used alone to treat Hodgkin lymphoma.
- Immunotherapy may be used to treat Hodgkin lymphoma that doesn't respond to treatment (refractory) or that returns after treatment (relapsed).
- Rituximab (Rituxan) is a targeted therapy widely used alone or in combination with chemotherapy to treat NLPHL
- A stem cell transplant destroys bone marrow then replaces it by adding healthy stem cells into your body. It may be an option for refractory or relapsed Hodgkin lymphoma.

4

Classic Hodgkin lymphoma (CHL)

This chapter presents the treatment options for classic Hodgkin lymphoma (CHL). CHL may be treated with only chemotherapy, or with both chemotherapy and radiation therapy. A stem cell transplant may be needed for CHL that doesn't respond to treatment.

Early CHL (stage I-II)

Stage I–II CHL may have certain features that make it harder to treat or that are known to lead to poorer outcomes. Your doctor may refer to these as "unfavorable" risk factors. These unfavorable risk factors include:

- B symptoms (unexplained high fevers, drenching night sweats, weight loss)
- A large ("bulky") tumor in your chest
- Cancerous lymph nodes larger than 10 cm
- High erythrocyte sedimentation rate (ESR)
- Having cancer in more than 3 areas

In order to plan treatment, doctors often group people with stage I–II CHL into one of 2 categories. **Low-risk** or favorable early disease means that the cancer doesn't have any of the risk factors listed above. **High-risk** or unfavorable early disease means that the cancer has one or more of the risk factors listed above.

There are 2 main approaches to treating early (stage I-II) CHL:

- Combination therapy (treatment with both chemotherapy and radiation therapy)
- Chemotherapy alone

The choice of approach is based on:

- Age
- Sex assigned at birth
- Family history of cancer or heart disease
- Other health problems
- The specific areas with cancer

Before final treatment decisions are made, it is recommended that a multidisciplinary team provides input. Multidisciplinary means that experts who specialize in different areas of cancer treatment are represented.

Low-risk, early CHL

Low-risk, early disease means that the cancer does not have any of the risk factors. Treatment begins with 2 cycles of chemotherapy with the ABVD regimen. After chemotherapy, you will have a PET/CT scan to see if the cancer improved. Further treatment depends on the results of the PET scan (the Deauville score).

Deauville score of 1 or 2

For a Deauville score of 1 or 2 after chemotherapy, both chemotherapy and combination therapy are options.

If chemotherapy alone is planned, 1 or 2 more cycles of ABVD is recommended. Having 2 cycles is preferred.

If combination therapy is planned, options include:

- Radiation therapy alone
- 1 cycle of ABVD and radiation therapy

Deauville score of 3
For a Deauville score of 3 after chemotherapy, both chemotherapy and combination therapy are options.

If chemotherapy alone is planned, 4 cycles of AVD (not ABVD) is recommended.

If combination therapy is planned, options include:

- Radiation therapy alone
- 2 cycles of ABVD and radiation therapy

Deauville score of 4
For a Deauville score of 4, having 2 more cycles of ABVD is often the next step. After finishing chemotherapy, you will have another PET scan. Further treatment depends on the results of the new (interim) Deauville score.

If the interim Deauville score is 1, 2, or 3, radiation therapy is recommended. If the interim Deauville score is 4 or 5, a biopsy is needed. If the biopsy is negative for lymphoma, radiation therapy is recommended. If the biopsy is positive, treatment for refractory CHL is recommended.

Deauville score of 5
If the Deauville score is 5 after 2 cycles of ABVD chemotherapy, a biopsy is needed before further treatment. If the biopsy is negative, the cancer is treated as if the Deauville score were 4 (see "Deauville score of 4" above). If the biopsy is positive, treatment for refractory CHL is recommended.

High-risk, early CHL

High-risk, early disease means that the cancer has 1 or more of the risk factors listed on the previous page. Treatment begins with 2 cycles of chemotherapy with the ABVD regimen. After chemotherapy, you will have a PET/CT scan to see if the cancer improved. Further treatment depends on the results of the PET scan (the Deauville score).

Deauville score of 1, 2, or 3
For a Deauville score of 1 to 3 after chemotherapy, both chemotherapy and combination therapy are options. If chemotherapy alone is planned, 4 cycles of AVD (not ABVD) are recommended. If combination therapy is planned, 2 cycles of ABVD and radiation therapy are recommended.

Deauville score of 4 or 5
For a Deauville score of 4 or 5 after chemotherapy, 2 cycles of chemotherapy with the escalated BEACOPP regimen is recommended. After finishing chemotherapy, you will have another PET scan. Further treatment depends on the results of the new (interim) Deauville score.

If the interim Deauville score is 1, 2, or 3, both chemotherapy and combination therapy are options. If chemotherapy alone is planned, 2 more cycles of escalated BEACOPP are recommended. If combination therapy is planned, radiation therapy is recommended.

If the interim Deauville score is 4 or 5, a biopsy is needed. If the biopsy is negative, radiation therapy is recommended. If the biopsy is positive, treatment for refractory CHL is recommended.

Advanced CHL (stage III–IV)

This section explains the recommended treatment options for CHL that has spread below the diaphragm, and possibly outside the lymphatic system.

Prognostic scores

Cancer researchers have developed a scoring system used to help guide treatment decisions for people with advanced CHL.

The risk factors below have been shown to contribute to poor treatment outcomes in people with stage III-IV CHL.

- Age 45 years or over
- Male sex assigned at birth
- Stage IV disease
- Albumin level below 4 g/dL
- A low hemoglobin level for your age and sex (commonly known as anemia)
- A high number of white blood cells in the blood (called leukocytosis)
- A low level of lymphocytes in the blood (called lymphocytopenia)

The score is calculated by adding the number of these risk factors that apply to you or your cancer. The total is called the International Prognostic Score (IPS).

Overview of treatment

Chemotherapy is always used to treat stage III and IV CHL. Radiation therapy may be added. The two preferred regimens used to treat advanced CHL are listed below.

- ABVD chemotherapy
- Brentuximab vedotin plus AVD chemotherapy

A third regimen that is used in some cases is escalated-dose BEACOPP. More information on these regimens and when each may be used is provided next.

ABVD chemotherapy

This treatment pathway is recommended for most people with stage III–IV CHL. Treatment begins with 2 cycles of chemotherapy with the ABVD regimen, followed by a PET/CT scan. Further treatment depends on the results of the PET scan (the Deauville score) and may include chemotherapy, radiation therapy, or both.

Deauville score of 1, 2, or 3

The next step is to have 4 cycles of AVD (not ABVD) chemotherapy. AVD chemotherapy does not include bleomycin. In some cases radiation therapy may also be used to treat high-risk areas. After chemotherapy, follow-up care begins.

Deauville score of 4 or 5

If the Deauville score is 4 or 5, switching to escalated BEACOPP chemotherapy for 3 cycles is recommended. Escalated BEACOPP is only an option for people under the age of 60.

After chemotherapy, you will have another PET/CT scan to see if the cancer improved.

Further treatment depends on the new (interim) Deauville score.

If the interim Deauville score is 1, 2, or 3, one more cycle of escalated BEACOPP is recommended. Radiation therapy may be given during the same time period.

If the interim Deauville score is 4 or 5, a biopsy is recommended. If the biopsy is negative for lymphoma, one more cycle of escalated BEACOPP is recommended. Radiation therapy may be given during the same time period. If the biopsy is positive, treatment for refractory (persistent) CHL is recommended.

Brentuximab vedotin and AVD

This regimen may be a good option for people who can't have bleomycin and for those with high-risk disease (IPS score of 4 or higher). It should not be used in people with nerve problems or damage (neuropathy). And, this regimen should be used with caution in people over the age of 60.

Treatment begins with 6 cycles of chemotherapy with brentuximab vedotin plus AVD. You will then have a PET/CT scan in order to restage the cancer. Your doctor may choose to do the PET/CT scan after only 2 cycles to help guide your care. Further treatment depends on the Deauville score. Regardless of Deauville score, radiation therapy may be used to treat high-risk areas.

Deauville score of 1, 2, or 3
If the Deauville score is 1, 2, or 3, no further chemotherapy is needed. You can begin follow-up care.

Deauville score of 4 or 5
If the Deauville score is 4 or 5, a biopsy is needed. If the biopsy is negative, you can begin follow-up care. If the biopsy is positive, treatment for refractory (persistent) CHL is recommended.

Escalated BEACOPP chemotherapy

This regimen may be a good option for some people under the age of 60 who have an IPS score of 4 or higher. Treatment begins with 2 cycles of chemotherapy with the escalated BEACOPP regimen. Then, you will have a PET/CT scan to restage the cancer. Further treatment depends on the Deauville score.

Deauville score of 1, 2, or 3
More chemotherapy is needed. One option is to continue escalated BEACOPP for 2 more cycles. Or, your doctor may recommend switching to either ABVD or AVD chemotherapy for 4 cycles. High-risk areas may also be treated with radiation therapy.

Deauville score of 4 or 5
A biopsy is needed. If the biopsy is positive, treatment for refractory (persistent) CHL is recommended.

If the biopsy is negative, continue escalated BEACOPP chemotherapy for 2 more cycles (bringing you to 4 cycles total). Next, a PET/CT scan is done to see if the cancer improved. Further treatment depends on the new (interim) Deauville score.

If the interim Deauville score is 1, 2, or 3, you will continue escalated BEACOPP chemotherapy for 2 more cycles. You may also have radiation therapy to high-risk areas.

If the interim Deauville score is 4 or 5, another biopsy is recommended. If the biopsy is negative, continue escalated BEACOPP chemotherapy for 2 more cycles. You may also have radiation therapy to high-risk areas. If the biopsy is positive, treatment for refractory (persistent) CHL is recommended.

Refractory CHL

Cancer that does not respond to treatment is called refractory. Refractory CHL is confirmed by biopsy. Treatment with systemic therapy is recommended for everyone with refractory CHL. It is called second-line therapy because it is given when initial (first-line) therapy does not work or stops working. Recommended second-line chemotherapy regimens are listed in **Guide 2.**

Guide 2 Second-line systemic therapy regimens
Brentuximab vedotin
Brentuximab vedotin and bendamustine
Brentuximab vedotin and nivolumab
DHAP (dexamethasone, cisplatin, high-dose cytarabine)
Gemcitabine, bendamustine, and vinorelbine
GVD (gemcitabine, vinorelbine, liposomal doxorubicin)
GVD and pembrolizumab
ICE (ifosfamide, carboplatin, etoposide)
ICE and brentuximab vedotin
ICE and nivolumab
IGEV (ifosfamide, gemcitabine, vinorelbine)
Pembrolizumab

After systemic therapy, the cancer will be restaged by doing another PET/CT scan. Further treatment is based on the Deauville score.

Deauville score of 1 to 3

An autologous stem cell transplant is recommended for everyone who can tolerate it. See page 25 for information on this procedure. Radiation therapy may be used to treat areas not previously treated with radiation. After the stem cell transplant (and radiation therapy, if you have it), there are two possibilities. If your doctor thinks the cancer is likely to return, maintenance therapy with brentuximab vedotin (Adcetris) will be considered. Otherwise, observation is recommended.

If you cannot have a stem cell transplant, taking a watch-and-wait approach (observation) is recommended. Radiation therapy may also be an option. You can then begin follow-up care.

Deauville score of 4 or 5

If the Deauville score is 4 or 5 after second-line systemic therapy, there are several options. The first option (stem cell transplant) will only be considered as the next treatment in those with a Deauville score of 4 after second-line systemic therapy.

Option 1: Stem cell transplant

An autologous stem cell transplant will be considered as the next treatment for those with a Deauville score of 4 after second-line systemic therapy. Radiation therapy may also be used. After the transplant, the need for further treatment depends on how likely the cancer is to return. If your doctor thinks the cancer is likely to return, maintenance therapy with brentuximab vedotin will be considered. Otherwise, observation is recommended.

Option 2: Radiation therapy
Radiation therapy alone is an option for those with a Deauville score of 4 or 5 after second-line therapy. If the cancer responds, a stem cell transplant will be considered. In this case, either an autologous or allogeneic transplant is an option.

Option 3: Systemic therapy
Another option for those with a Deauville score of 4 or 5 after second-line therapy is more systemic therapy. Radiation therapy may also be given. Options for systemic therapy include second-line regimens that you didn't already receive (**see Guide 2**). If the cancer responds, a stem cell transplant will be considered. In this case, either an autologous or allogeneic transplant is an option.

CHL in older adults

While CHL can often be cured in younger adults, treatment outcomes for older adults are not as good. People over 60 often have other, sometimes serious, health problems. They may also not be able to do certain daily tasks and activities. The cancer itself also tends to have different features in older adults. This can make it harder to treat.

Like in younger adults, the main treatment for CHL in older adults is chemotherapy. However, the standard chemotherapy regimens for CHL are too harsh and may be dangerous to use in older adults. For example, most of the chemotherapy regimens used to treat CHL in younger adults include the drug bleomycin (Blenoxane). Bleomycin can damage the lungs and cause a disease called pulmonary fibrosis. Pulmonary fibrosis is a buildup of scar tissue in the lungs. This buildup makes it hard to breathe and causes other side effects. Older adults with CHL may not be able to tolerate bleomycin. If used, it should not be given for more than 2 cycles.

There isn't a lot of research on alternatives to standard treatments for older patients. The goal is to find the most effective treatment that will cause the least amount of harm. Your doctor will consider your overall health, the features of the cancer, and the harshness of a chemotherapy regimen when recommending a treatment option.

The regimens in **Guide 3** on the next page are likely to be less harmful to older adults with CHL than standard regimens.

Older adults with CHL are more likely to have:

- ✓ B symptoms
- ✓ Other health problems
- ✓ The Epstein-Barr virus
- ✓ A subtype of CHL called mixed cellularity Hodgkin lymphoma (MCHL)

Unfortunately, treatment outcomes for older adults with CHL are usually poor, even if one of these milder regimens is used. For this reason, joining a clinical trial is recommended if one is available to you. If your doctor feels that you should not have any chemotherapy, treatment with radiation therapy alone is an option.

Guide 3
Treatment options for older adults with CHL

Stage I-II low-risk CHL

- **Preferred option:** 2 cycles of ABVD or AVD. May be followed by 2 cycles of AVD and radiation therapy.
- 4 cycles of CHOP + radiation therapy

Stage I-II high-risk CHL and stage III-IV CHL

- 2 cycles of ABVD or AVD, followed by a PET scan. If the scan is negative, 4 cycles of AVD is recommended. If the scan is positive, treatment is individualized.
- Chemotherapy with brentuximab vedotin followed by AVD. If good results, may be followed by more brentuximab vedotin.
- Chemotherapy with brentuximab vedotin and dacarbazine
- 6 cycles of CHOP chemotherapy, with or without radiation therapy

Refractory or relapsed CHL - Options for palliative therapy

- Chemotherapy with bendamustine
- Chemotherapy with brentuximab vedotin
- Radiation therapy
- Immunotherapy with nivolumab (Opdivo) or pembrolizumab (Keytruda)

Key points

Early CHL (stage I-II)

- Stage I–II CHL may have features that make it harder to treat or that are known to lead to poorer outcomes. Treatment is based in part on whether the cancer has any of these risk factors.
- The risk factors include large (bulky) tumors in your lymph nodes or chest, B symptoms, a fast erythrocyte sedimentation rate, and having cancer in more than 3 groups of lymph nodes.
- There are two main approaches for the initial treatment of CHL: chemotherapy and combination therapy (chemotherapy and radiation therapy).
- It is important to have another PET/CT scan within 3 months of finishing treatment. If the PET/CT finds no signs of cancer, you can begin follow-up care.

Advanced CHL (stage III-IV)

- Chemotherapy is always used to treat stage III and IV CHL. Radiation therapy may be given in addition to chemotherapy.
- The two preferred regimens used to treat advanced CHL are ABVD chemotherapy and brentuximab vedotin plus AVD chemotherapy.
- A third regimen that is used in some cases is escalated-dose BEACOPP.

CHL in older adults

- While CHL is often curable in younger adults, treatment outcomes for older adults are not as good.
- The chemotherapy regimens for CHL are too harsh and may be dangerous to use in older adults.
- There are milder chemotherapy regimens that are likely to be less harmful to older adults. Joining a clinical trial is also recommended.

Refractory CHL

- An autologous stem cell transplant is recommended for CHL that doesn't respond to treatment (refractory) or that returns after treatment (relapsed).

5

Nodular lymphocyte-predominant Hodgkin lymphoma (NLPHL)

NLPHL is a rare type of Hodgkin lymphoma. It is often slow-growing and may return long after treatment (relapse). However, more treatment is not always needed for relapsed NLPHL. Over time, NLPHL can transform into an aggressive type of non-Hodgkin lymphoma.

About NLPHL

NLPHL is usually found at an early stage. It doesn't tend to have any high-risk features when it is diagnosed. NLPHL can transform into an aggressive type of non-Hodgkin lymphoma called diffuse large B-cell lymphoma (DLBCL).

NLPHL is more likely to transform into an aggressive B-cell lymphoma if any of the following are found at the time of diagnosis:

- Large tumor(s) (the medical term for this is "bulky disease")
- Cancer below the diaphragm
- Cancer in the spleen

Overview of treatment

The three main treatments for NLPHL are:

- Radiation therapy
- Chemotherapy
- Targeted therapy with rituximab (Rituxan)

Depending on the cancer stage, the treatments may be used alone or combined. Treatment of NLPHL depends in part on the following:

- Whether the lymph nodes with cancer are large (bulky)
- Whether the cancer is only above the diaphragm (stage I–II) or whether it has spread below the diaphragm (stage III–IV)
- If the cancer is in only in 2 groups of lymph nodes above the diaphragm (stage II), treatment also depends on whether the lymph node groups with cancer are next to each other ("contiguous"). If they aren't, it is called "non-contiguous" disease.

Initial treatment

This section describes the initial treatment options for NLPHL, according to stage.

Stage IA and IIA

Most stage IA and IIA tumors are small (not bulky). Radiation therapy is recommended to treat these small, early-stage tumors. Some people with stage IA NLPHL may be able to safely skip radiation therapy. This may be the case if cancer was found in only one lymph node that was totally removed. In this situation, while radiation therapy is preferred, having no further treatment is an option.

While uncommon, stage IA and IIA tumors can be large (bulky). Stage IIA NLPHL may also be non-contiguous. This means that cancer is in 2 groups of lymph nodes above the diaphragm, but the groups are not next to each other. Treatment with both systemic therapy (chemotherapy plus rituximab) and radiation therapy is recommended for bulky stage IA and bulky or non-contiguous stage IIA NLPHL.

Radiation therapy alone may be an option for a small number of people with stage IIA non-contiguous disease.

Stage IB and IIB

Treatment with both systemic therapy (chemotherapy plus rituximab) and radiation therapy is recommended for stage IB and stage IIB NLPHL. Radiation therapy alone may be an option for a small number of people with stage IB disease.

Guide 4 lists the most common systemic therapy regimens used to treat NLPHL. When used in combination with radiation therapy, chemotherapy is generally only given for 2 to 4 months.

Stage III–IV

The initial treatment options for stage III–IV (advanced) NLPHL are listed below.

- Observation (if you do not have symptoms)
- Chemotherapy plus rituximab, and possibly also radiation therapy
- Rituximab alone
- Radiation therapy alone to relieve symptoms caused by the cancer

After finishing treatment, expect to have a positron emission tomography/computed tomography (PET/CT) scan to learn if the cancer improved. This is called restaging. If the cancer improves but you are still having symptoms, radiation therapy is recommended (if you haven't already had it). If the cancer improves and you do not have symptoms, you do not need more treatment. See *Part 6: When treatment is over.*

If the cancer does not improve or worsens, see the next page.

Guide 4 Commonly used first-line systemic therapy regimens for NLPHL
ABVD (doxorubicin, bleomycin, vinblastine, dacarbazine) + rituximab
CHOP (cyclophosphamide, doxorubicin, vincristine, prednisone) + rituximab
CVbP (cyclophosphamide, vinblastine, prednisolone) + rituximab
Rituximab alone **(an option for stage III-IV NLPHL)**

Refractory or relapsed NLPHL

Cancer that does not respond to initial treatment is called refractory. Cancer that returns after a cancer-free period is called relapsed.

Over time, NLPHL can turn into a fast-growing type of non-Hodgkin lymphoma called DLBCL. For refractory or relapsed NLPHL, a biopsy to learn if the cancer has transformed is recommended. This is needed because B-cell lymphoma is managed differently than NLPHL. The cancer type is confirmed by removing samples of one or more tumors and testing them in a lab.

If the biopsy is negative and you don't have any symptoms, observation is recommended.

If the biopsy confirms that the cancer has transformed, see the NCCN Guidelines for Patients: Diffuse Large B-cell Lymphoma.

If the biopsy confirms NLPHL, the cancer has not transformed. In this case, there are several options. NLPHL can be very slow-growing. Treatment is not always needed. Treatment decisions should be based on your general health and the features of the cancer. There isn't a "best" way to treat refractory or relapsed NLPHL. If treatment is needed, options include:

- Systemic therapy with rituximab alone. Some people may continue treatment with rituximab alone for 2 years. This is called maintenance therapy.
- Second-line systemic therapy with rituximab and chemotherapy. **See Guide 5.**
- Radiation therapy and second-line systemic therapy
- Radiation therapy alone

Guide 5 **Second-line and subsequent systemic therapy regimens for NLPHL**
Rituximab + bendamustine
Rituximab + DHAP (dexamethasone, cisplatin, high-dose cytarabine)
Rituximab + ICE (ifosfamide, carboplatin, etoposide)
Rituximab + IGEV (ifosfamide, gemcitabine, vinorelbine)
If not previously used, the following first-line systemic therapy regimens are also options: • Rituximab + ABVD (doxorubicin, bleomycin, vinblastine, dacarbazine) • Rituximab + CHOP (cyclophosphamide, doxorubicin, vincristine, prednisone) • Rituximab + CVbP (cyclophosphamide, vinblastine, prednisolone)

Key points

- NLPHL is a rare type of Hodgkin lymphoma. It is usually found at an early stage. It does not often have high-risk features when found.
- NLPHL can transform into an aggressive type of non-Hodgkin lymphoma called diffuse large B-cell lymphoma (DLBCL).

Stage I-II NLPHL

- Radiation therapy is the preferred treatment for most non-bulky stage IA and IIA NLPHLs.
- Initial treatment with both systemic therapy (chemotherapy plus rituximab) and radiation therapy is recommended for:
  - Bulky stage IA NLPHL
  - Bulky or non-contiguous stage IIA NLPHL
  - Stage IB and IIB NLPHL
  - Radiation therapy alone may be an option for some people with stage IIA non-contiguous NLPHL and stage IB NLPHL.

Stage III-IV NLPHL

- Initial treatment options include:
  - Observation (if you do not have symptoms)
  - Chemotherapy plus rituximab, and possibly also radiation therapy
  - Rituximab alone
  - Radiation therapy alone to relieve symptoms

Refractory or relapsed NLPHL

- A biopsy to learn if the cancer has transformed into DLBCL is recommended for refractory or relapsed NLPHL.
- If the biopsy confirms NLPHL, options may include:
  - Observation
  - Systemic therapy with rituximab alone, (2 years of maintenance therapy may follow)
  - Second-line systemic therapy with rituximab and chemotherapy
  - Radiation therapy and second-line systemic therapy
  - Radiation therapy alone

6

When treatment is over

Hodgkin lymphoma can usually be cured. But, its treatment can cause serious health problems—including other cancers—down the line. When treatment is over, it is important to see an oncologist who understands the unique risks and health issues faced by Hodgkin lymphoma survivors.

Good to know

There isn't a "one-size-fits-all" care plan that all Hodgkin lymphoma survivors should follow after treatment. The types of follow-up tests you should have—and how often you should have them—should be based on your specific cancer circumstances. This includes:

- ✓ Your age
- ✓ The cancer stage when you were diagnosed
- ✓ Your social habits
- ✓ Your treatment history

The first 5 years

During the first 5 years after treatment, it is important to monitor for the return of Hodgkin lymphoma. The recommended care during this time is explained below.

Physical exams

Physical exams are an important part of follow-up care. They are given more often in the years right after treatment, and then spaced farther apart in later years. During the first 1 to 2 years, a physical exam is recommended every 3 to 6 months. They are then given every 6 to 12 months until 5 years after treatment. Annual (yearly) exams are recommended after that.

Blood tests

There is no recommended schedule for bloodwork in the first 5 years after treatment. Your doctor may order blood tests at the time of your physical exams, or may only order them if relapse is suspected.

Blood tests your doctor may order include a complete blood count (CBC), erythrocyte sedimentation rate (ESR), and chemistry profile. An ESR is usually only needed if your initial ESR was high. If you had radiation therapy to the neck, a thyroid-stimulating hormone (TSH) test is recommended at least once a year.

Imaging tests

During the first 2 years after treatment, you may have a computed tomography (CT) scan of your neck, chest, abdomen, and pelvis every 6 months. Or, your doctor may only order a CT scan if you have symptoms, or if there are other reasons to suspect the cancer has returned. A contrast agent should be used during any follow-up CT scans. After 2 years,

CT scans are given as needed, especially for NLPHL, which can return long after treatment.

You may need a PET/CT if the results of your last PET/CT suggested a poor response to treatment. However, having PET scans on a regular basis to monitor for the return of Hodgkin lymphoma is not recommended.

Survivorship counseling

There are both short- and long-term health effects of Hodgkin lymphoma and its treatment. It is important to be aware of the unique risks and health issues faced by Hodgkin lymphoma survivors. Ask your doctor about:

- What to expect now that treatment is over
- Fertility and family planning issues
- The importance of leading a healthy lifestyle after cancer treatment
- Your increased risk of other cancers (eg, skin cancer and breast cancer) and steps to help prevent them (eg, breast self-exams)
- The importance of taking care of your mental and emotional health
- Survivorship support groups or clinics

Survivorship counseling

Hodgkin lymphoma survivors are encouraged to undergo counseling on survivorship, including long-term treatment effects, preventing new cancers, and healthy behaviors. Ask your doctor about survivorship clinics near you.

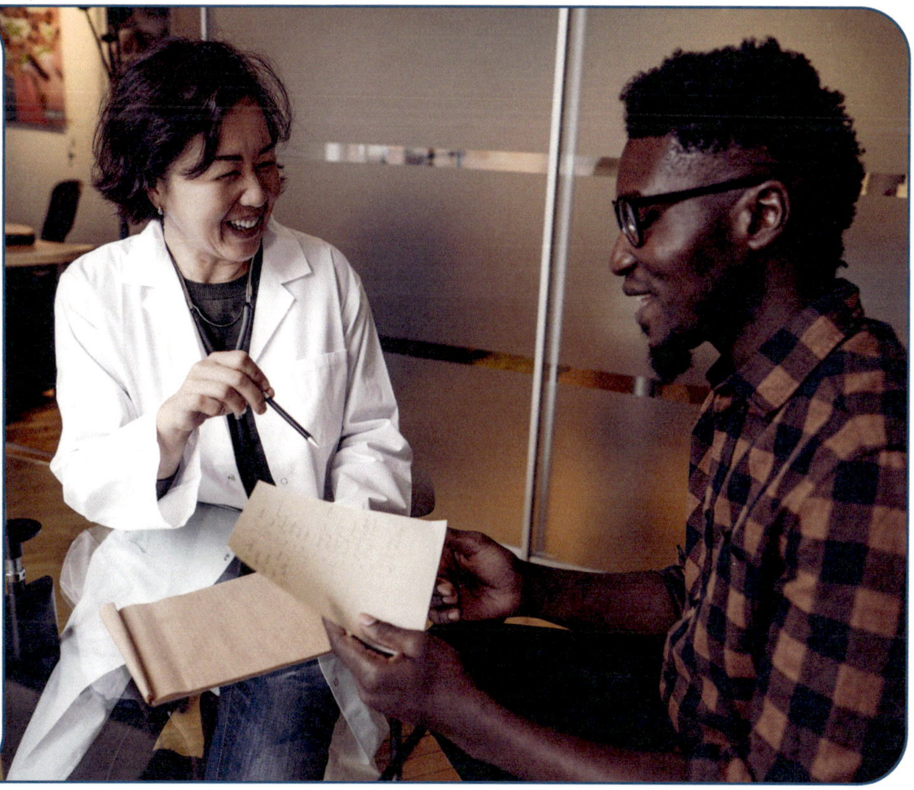

For more information on cancer survivorship, the following are available at NCCN.org/patientguidelines and on the NCCN Patient Guides for Cancer app:

- *Survivorship Care for Healthy Living*
- *Survivorship Care for Cancer-Related Late and Long-term Effects*

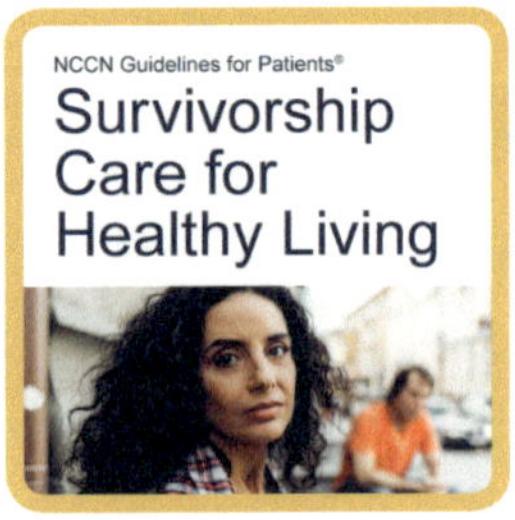

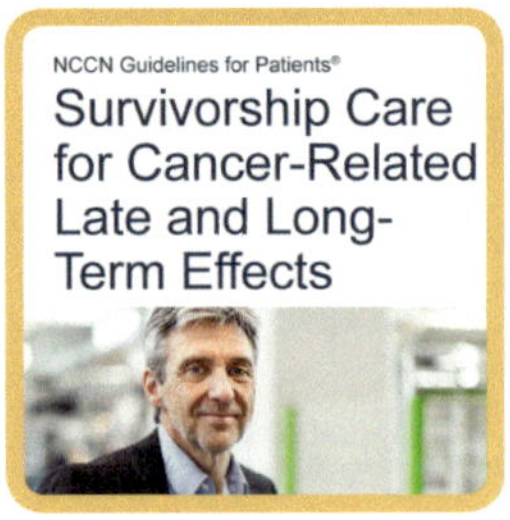

These resources address topics relevant to survivors of Hodgkin lymphoma, including:

- Anxiety, depression, and distress
- Cognitive dysfunction
- Fatigue
- Pain
- Sexual problems
- Sleep problems
- Healthy lifestyles
- Immunizations
- Employment, insurance, and disability

Try to remember that not every new symptom means that your cancer has returned. Make sure to establish care with a primary care doctor.

share with us.

Take our survey.
And help make the
NCCN Guidelines for Patients
better for everyone!

NCCN.org/patients/comments

Long-term follow-up care

Side effects of Hodgkin lymphoma and its treatment can start years after treatment. These are called "late" side effects. The most serious late effects that long-term Hodgkin survivors experience are:

- Other cancers
- Heart disease
- Underactive thyroid (hypothyroidism)
- Fertility issues

The longer you are monitored after finishing treatment, the more likely you are to experience some of these side effects. The long-term care you should receive is described next.

Physical exams

Physical exams continue to be an important part of follow-up care. Beginning in the sixth year after treatment, you should have a physical exam once a year. Your doctor should closely monitor changes in your blood pressure. Any signs of heart damage or disease should be noted and promptly managed.

Blood tests

You should have a CBC and a chemistry profile once a year beginning in the sixth year after treatment. If your neck was treated with radiation, continue to have your TSH level measured at least once a year.

Due to the increased risk of heart damage or disease over time, extra bloodwork to test for lipid disorders and diabetes is needed after 5 years. Lipids are fats that your body uses for energy. Cholesterol is a lipid. You should have

Physical exams

Physical exams are needed more often right after treatment and then spaced farther apart. Starting in the sixth year after treatment, a physical exam is recommended once per year.

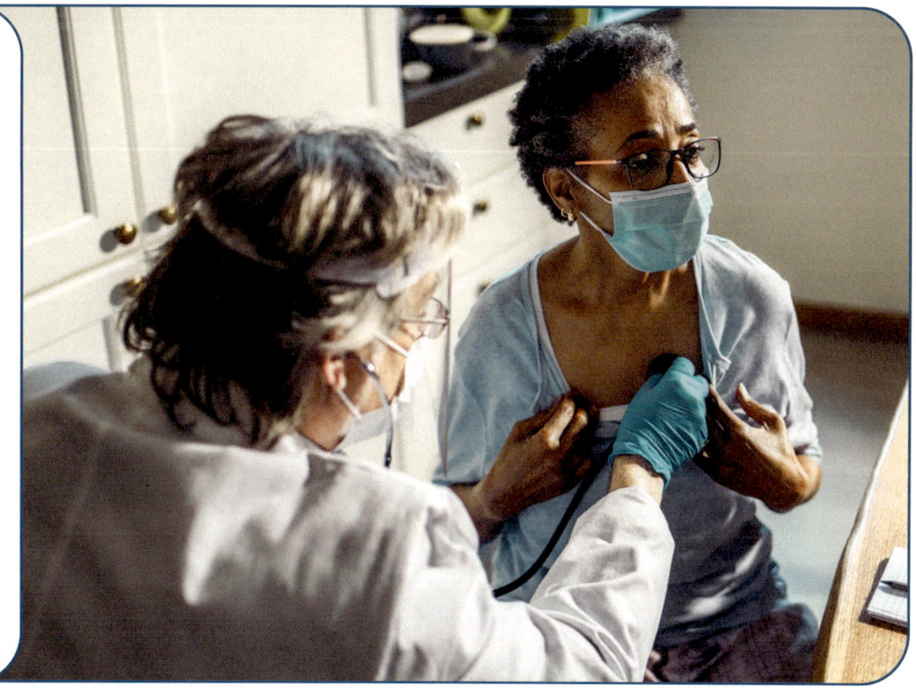

a test called a lipids panel twice per year. A lipids panel typically measures your:

- Total cholesterol level
- Triglyceride level
- The levels of "good" (HDL) and "bad" (LDL) cholesterol

Glucose—a simple sugar—is your body's main source of energy. A fasting glucose test measures the amount of glucose in your blood. If your blood glucose levels are high, it could be a sign of diabetes. If your blood glucose levels are low, it could be a sign of hypothyroidism. A fasting glucose test is recommended once a year beginning in the sixth year after finishing treatment.

Thyroid problems

The thyroid is a small, butterfly-shaped gland in the front of the neck. About half of Hodgkin lymphoma survivors who had radiation therapy to the neck or upper chest have thyroid problems later in life. The most common problem is hypothyroidism, in which the thyroid gland doesn't make enough thyroid hormone. Weight gain, constipation, dry skin, and sensitivity to cold temperatures are symptoms of an underactive thyroid.

Your doctor should do a careful thyroid examination during your annual physical exam. Thyroid function tests should also be done at least once a year to rule out hypothyroidism, especially in people who had radiation therapy to the neck.

Vaccines

Everyone should continue to get the influenza vaccine (the "flu shot") every year, and other vaccines as needed. This includes the COVID-19 vaccine. NCCN offers more information on COVID-19 at NCCN.org/covid-19.

Thyroid exams

About half of Hodgkin lymphoma survivors who had radiation therapy to the neck or upper chest have thyroid problems later in life. A careful thyroid examination is an important part of your annual physical exam.

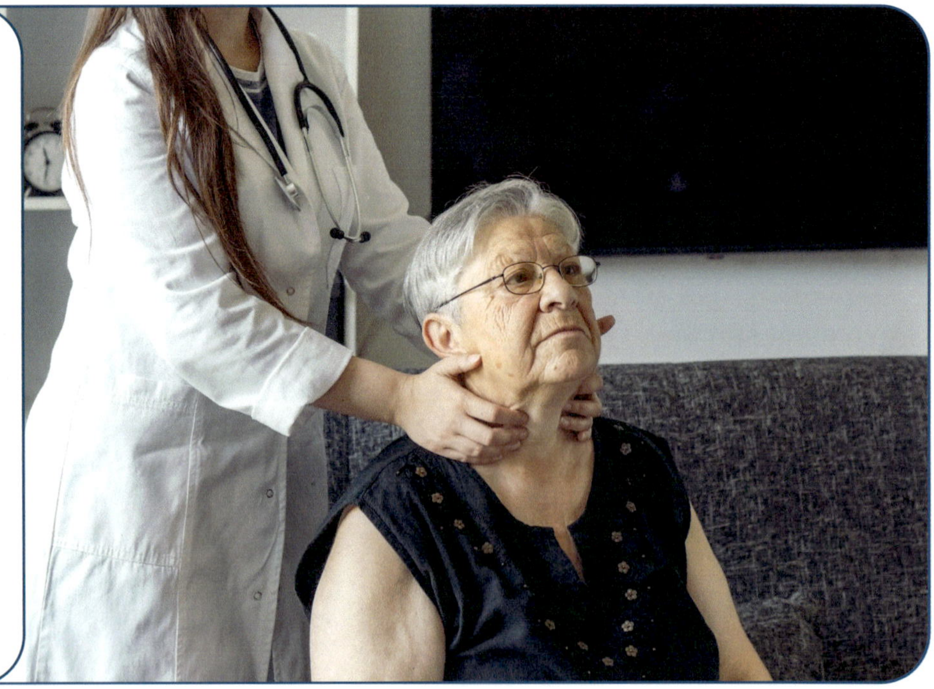

People treated with radiation therapy to the spleen or who had a splenectomy should be re-vaccinated against pneumonia, meningitis, and Haemophilus influenzae type B ("Hib") 5 to 7 years after treatment.

Screening for other cancers

Anyone who has had Hodgkin lymphoma is at risk of getting other types of cancer. This is especially true if radiation therapy was used as part of first-line treatment. These "secondary cancers" often occur more than 10 years after finishing treatment for Hodgkin lymphoma. Lung cancer and breast cancer are the most common secondary cancers in Hodgkin lymphoma survivors. Skin cancers can also occur in areas treated with radiation.

Those assigned female at birth who had radiation therapy to the chest or armpit area should start screening for breast cancer 8 years after finishing treatment, or at age 40 (whichever comes first).

Those assigned female at birth who had radiation therapy to the chest between age 10 and age 30 should be screened with both mammography and breast magnetic resonance imaging (MRI). NCCN experts also encourage doing monthly breast self-exams, and having a breast exam by a health care professional once a year. Your doctor may also refer you to a breast specialist.

Screening for cervical, colorectal, endometrial, lung, and prostate cancer is also recommended. Screening should follow the recommendations of NCCN and the American Cancer Society (ACS).

Heart disease

Hodgkin lymphoma survivors have a higher long-term risk of diseases that affect the heart or blood vessels. This is called heart disease

Breast cancer screening

Many Hodgkin lymphoma survivors get breast cancer later in life. Those who had radiation therapy to the chest or armpit area should start screening for breast cancer 8 to 10 years after finishing treatment, or at age 40 (whichever comes first).

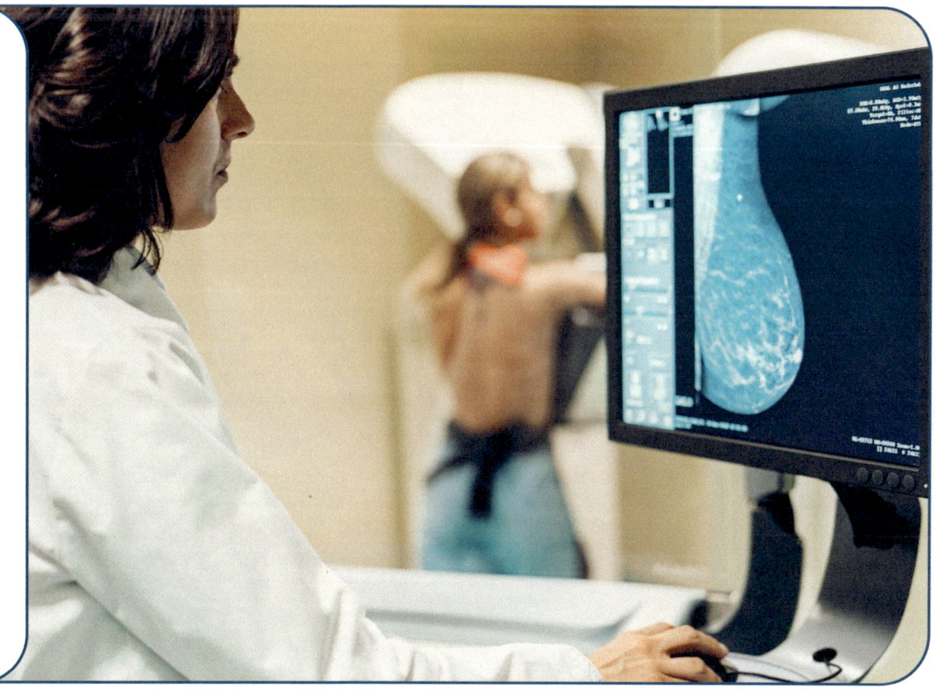

or cardiovascular disease. Symptoms of heart disease can start at any age, but damage to the heart or blood vessels is usually found more than 5 to 10 years after finishing treatment.

The biggest risk factors for developing heart disease in Hodgkin lymphoma survivors are:

- Treatment with radiation therapy to the area between the lungs
- Treatment with chemotherapy medicines called anthracyclines.

Doxorubicin is an anthracycline used in some chemotherapy regimens widely used to treat Hodgkin lymphoma, including ABVD and escalated BEACOPP.

Everyone treated for Hodgkin lymphoma should have their blood pressure taken at least once a year and the levels closely monitored, even if there are no symptoms of heart disease.

Your doctor may order an exercise stress test or heart ultrasound (echocardiogram) when you are done treatment. If you had radiation therapy to the neck, your doctor may also order an ultrasound of your carotid artery. The goal is to get a baseline (starting) measurement of your heart health. The testing may then be repeated every 10 years. The results will be compared to your baseline results.

Exercise stress test

In order to monitor for signs of heart disease, you may have an exercise stress test every 10 years after finishing treatment.

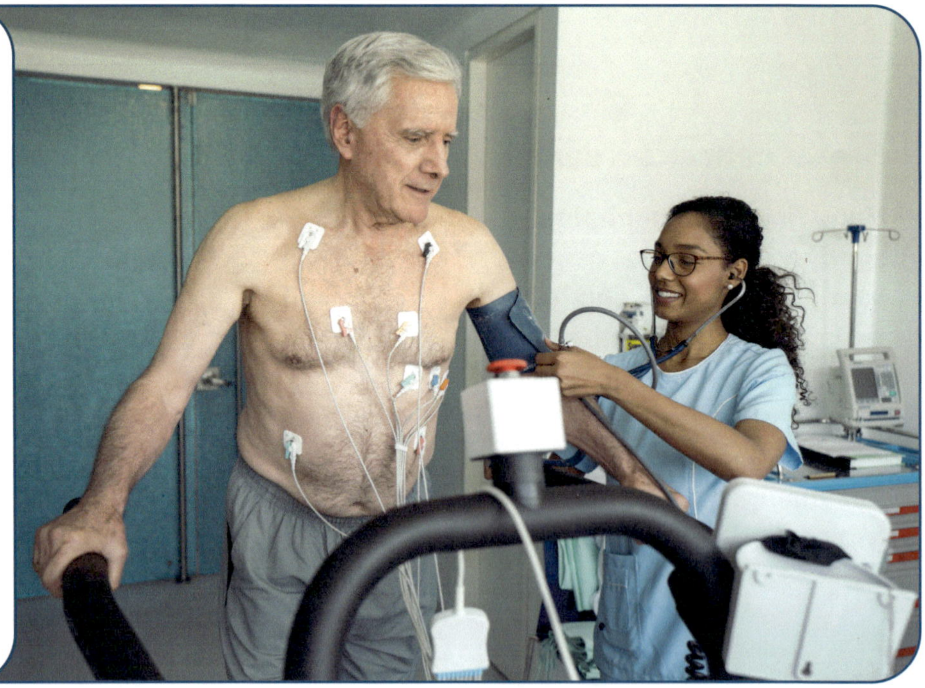

Key points

- Treatment for Hodgkin lymphoma can cause other health problems later in life.
- The most serious late effects that survivors experience are other cancers, heart disease, hypothyroidism, and fertility issues.
- Follow-up testing should be personalized and based on your specific cancer circumstances.
- Ask your doctor for a summary of your cancer treatment history and related health risks.

The first 5 years after treatment

- During the first 1 to 2 years, a physical exam is recommended every 3 to 6 months. An exam is then given every 6 to 12 months through the fifth year.
- During the first 2 years after treatment, you may have CT imaging every 6 months. Or, your doctor may only order a CT scan if recurrence is suspected.
- After 2 years, CT scans are given as needed, especially for NLPHL, which can return long after treatment.

Long-term follow-up care

- Beginning in the sixth year after treatment, a physical exam is recommended once a year.
- A CBC, chemistry profile, and fasting glucose test are recommended once a year beginning in the sixth year after treatment. If your neck was treated with radiation, your TSH level will be continue to be checked at least once a year. A lipids panel is recommended twice per year.
- Hypothyroidism is a common late effect of Hodgkin lymphoma treatment with radiation therapy. Symptoms include weight gain, constipation, dry skin, and sensitivity to cold temperatures.
- The risk of secondary cancers is increased in Hodgkin lymphoma survivors. Lung cancer and breast cancer are the most common secondary cancers.
- Those who had radiation therapy to the chest or armpit area should start screening mammography 8 years after treatment or at age 40 (whichever comes first).
- Both mammography and MRI are recommended for those who had radiation therapy to the chest between age 10 and 30.
- Screening for cervical, colorectal, endometrial, lung, skin, and prostate cancer is recommended.
- Hodgkin lymphoma survivors have a higher long-term risk of heart disease. Your blood pressure will be checked at least once a year. Additional testing may be ordered after treatment and repeated every 10 years.

7
Making treatment decisions

It is important to be comfortable with the cancer treatment you choose. This choice starts with having an open and honest conversation with your care team.

It's your choice

In shared decision-making, you and your care team share information, discuss the options, and agree on a treatment plan. It starts with an open and honest conversation between you and your team.

Treatment decisions are very personal. What is important to you may not be important to someone else. Some things that may play a role in your decision-making:

- What you want and how that might differ from what others want
- Your religious and spiritual beliefs
- Your feelings about certain treatments
- Your feelings about pain or side effects
- Cost of treatment, travel to treatment centers, and time away from school or work
- Quality of life and length of life
- How active you are and the activities that are important to you

Think about what you want from treatment. Discuss openly the risks and benefits of specific treatments and procedures. Weigh options and share concerns with your doctor. If you take the time to build a relationship with your team, it will help you feel supported when considering options and making treatment decisions.

Second opinion

It is normal to want to start treatment as soon as possible. While cancer should not be ignored, there is time to have another cancer care provider review your test results and suggest a treatment plan. This is called getting a second opinion, and it's a normal part of cancer care. Even doctors get second opinions!

Things you can do to prepare:

- Check with your insurance company about its rules on second opinions. There may be out-of-pocket costs to see doctors who are not part of your insurance plan.
- Make plans to have copies of all your records sent to the doctor you will see for your second opinion.

Support groups

Many people diagnosed with cancer find support groups to be helpful. Support groups often include people at different stages of treatment. Some people may be newly diagnosed, while others may be finished with treatment. If your hospital or community doesn't have support groups for people with cancer, check out the websites listed in this book. If you are an adolescent or young adult (an "AYA"), ask your care team about AYA-specific support groups.

Questions to ask

Possible questions to ask your cancer care team are listed on the following pages. Feel free to use these or come up with your own. Be clear about your goals for treatment and find out what to expect from treatment.

Questions about cancer testing

1. What tests will I have?
2. Do the tests have any risks?
3. Will my insurance pay for all of the tests you are recommending?
4. Do I need to do anything to prepare for testing?
5. Should I bring someone with me to the appointments?
6. Where do I go for testing, and how long will it take?
7. If any of the tests will hurt, what will you do to make me comfortable?
8. How soon will I know the results and who will explain them to me?
9. Is there an online portal with my test results?
10. Can we discuss my options for receiving test results?

Questions about treatment options

1. What are my treatment options?
2. Is a clinical trial an option for me?
3. How long do I have to decide about treatment? What will happen if I do nothing?
4. Are you suggesting options other than what NCCN recommends? If yes, why?
5. How do my age, sex, overall health, and other factors affect my options?
6. What if I am pregnant, or planning to become pregnant?
7. Does any option offer a cure or long-term cancer control?
8. How do I get a second opinion?
9. Are there support services (eg, patient navigators; support groups) available to me during treatment?
10. Do I need an advanced directive? When and how do I prepare an advanced directive?

Questions about side effects

1. What are the possible complications and side effects of treatment?
2. Does the cancer itself cause any side effects?
3. Which side effects are most common and how long do they usually last?
4. Which side effects are serious or life-threatening?
5. Are there any long-term or permanent side effects?
6. What symptoms should I report right away, and who do I contact?
7. What can I do to prevent or relieve the side effects of treatment?
8. Do any medications worsen side effects?
9. Do any side effects lessen or worsen in severity over time?
10. Will you stop or change treatment if there are serious side effects?

Resources

American Association for Cancer Research (AACR)
aacr.org/patients-caregivers/cancer/hodgkin-lymphoma/

American Cancer Society
cancer.org/cancer/hodgkin-lymphoma.html

Be The Match
bethematch.org

Blood & Marrow Transplant Information Network
bmtinfonet.org

Canadian Cancer Society
cancer.ca/en/cancer-information/cancer-types/hodgkin-lymphoma/what-is-hodgkin-lymphoma

Cancer.Net
cancer.net/cancer-types/lymphoma-hodgkin

CancerCare
Cancercare.org

Cancer Hope Network
cancerhopenetwork.org

Cancer Support Community
cancersupportcommunity.org

Elephants and Tea
elephantsandtea.com

Leukaemia Foundation
leukaemia.org.au/blood-cancer-information/types-of-blood-cancer/lymphoma/hodgkin-lymphoma

Livestrong
livestrong.org

Lymphoma Research Foundation
lymphoma.org/understanding-lymphoma/aboutlymphoma/hl

National Bone Marrow Transplant Link
nbmtLINK.org

National Cancer Institute (NCI)
cancer.gov/types/lymphoma

National Coalition for Cancer Survivorship
canceradvocacy.org

NCCN Patient and Caregiver Resources
NCCN.org/patients

PAN Foundation
panfoundation.org

Stupid Cancer
stupidcancer.org

The Leukemia & Lymphoma Society (LLS)
LLS.org/PatientSupport

U.S. National Library of Medicine Clinical Trials Database
clinicaltrials.gov

Young Adult Cancer Connection (YACC)
yacancerconnection.org

Words to know

abdomen
The area of the body between the chest and pelvis. Contains the pancreas, stomach, intestines, liver, gallbladder, and other organs.

allogeneic stem cell transplant
A cancer treatment that replaces abnormal blood stem cells with healthy donor cells. Also called allogeneic hematopoietic cell transplant (HCT).

autologous stem cell transplant
A treatment that destroys your bone marrow then rebuilds it with your healthy stem cells. Also called high-dose therapy with autologous stem cell rescue (HDT/ASCR).

B symptoms
High fevers, heavy night sweats, and fast weight loss without dieting caused by Hodgkin lymphoma.

biopsy
Removal of small amounts of tissue or fluid to be tested for disease.

blood chemistry profile
A lab test of the amount of 8 chemicals in a sample of blood.

body plethysmograph
A test done in a small room with a small tube to measure how much air is in your lungs after inhaling or exhaling.

bone marrow
Soft, sponge-like tissue in the center of most bones where blood cells are made.

bone marrow aspiration
A procedure that removes a liquid bone marrow sample to test for disease.

bone marrow biopsy
Removal of a small amount of solid bone and bone marrow to test for disease.

cancer stage
A rating of the extent of cancer in the body.

chemotherapy
The use of medicines that stop the growth of cancer cells.

classic Hodgkin lymphoma (CHL)
The most common type of Hodgkin lymphoma.

clinical trial
A type of research that studies how well medical tests and treatments work in people.

complete blood count (CBC)
A test of the number of blood cells in a sample.

comprehensive metabolic panel
Tests of about 14 chemicals in your blood.

computed tomography (CT)
A test that uses x-rays from many angles to make pictures of areas inside the body.

contiguous lymphoma
Lymphoma in which the lymph nodes with cancer are next to each other.

contrast
A substance put into your body to make clearer pictures during imaging tests.

core needle biopsy
The removal of a tissue sample with a wide needle for examination under a microscope. Also called core biopsy.

Deauville scale
A rating by doctors of treatment response based on comparing the uptake of a radiotracer by cancer sites to two other sites.

diaphragm
The thin muscle below the lungs and heart that helps a person to breathe.

diffuse large B-cell lymphoma (DLBCL)
A common type of B-cell non-Hodgkin lymphoma that is usually fast-growing.

echocardiogram
A test that uses sound waves to make pictures of the heart.

ejection fraction
The amount of blood pumped out of the left side of your heart.

erythrocyte sedimentation rate (ESR)
A test for inflammation based on how much clear liquid is at the top of a tube of blood after one hour.

excisional biopsy
A procedure that removes entire lymph nodes to test for cancer cells.

external beam radiation therapy (EBRT)
Radiation therapy received from a machine outside the body.

fatigue
Severe tiredness despite getting enough sleep that limits one's ability to function.

fertility specialist
An expert who helps people have children.

fine-needle aspiration (FNA)
Use of a thin needle to remove fluid or tissue from the body to test for disease.

gas diffusion test
A test that uses harmless gas to measure how much a person can breathe out.

general anesthesia
A drug-induced, sleep-like state for pain relief.

Hodgkin lymphoma
A cancer that starts in a type of white blood cell (lymphocyte). Reed-Sternberg cells are present.

immune system
The body's natural defense against infection and disease.

immunohistochemistry (IHC)
A test of cancer cells to find specific cell traits involved in abnormal cell growth.

involved-site radiation therapy (ISRT)
Treatment with high-energy rays (radiation) that is delivered to lymph nodes and nearby sites with cancer.

lactate dehydrogenase
A protein that helps to make energy in cells.

liver
An organ that removes waste from the blood and helps to digest food.

liver function test
Test that measures chemicals in the blood that are made or processed by the liver.

local anesthesia
A drug-induced loss of feeling in a small area of the body.

lung function test
A test used to measure how well the lungs work. Also called pulmonary function test.

lymph
A clear fluid containing white blood cells.

lymphatic system
The tissues and organs that produce, store, and carry white blood cells that fight infections and other diseases.

lymph node
Small groups of disease-fighting cells located throughout the body.

lymphocyte
A type of immune cell that is made in the bone marrow and is found in the blood and in lymph tissue.

mediastinum
The area of the chest between the lungs.

noncontiguous lymphoma
Lymphoma in which the lymph nodes containing cancer are on the same side of the diaphragm, but are not next to each other.

positron emission tomography/computed tomography (PET/CT) scan
A procedure that uses two types of imaging techniques (PET and CT) to create detailed pictures of areas inside the body.

positron emission tomography (PET) scan
A test that uses a small amount of radioactive glucose (sugar) and a scanner to see where glucose is being used in the body.

spleen
An organ that is part of the lymphatic system and helps protect the body from disease. It is located on the left side of the abdomen near the stomach.

Let us know what you think!

Please take a moment to complete an online survey about the NCCN Guidelines for Patients.

NCCN.org/patients/response

NCCN Contributors

This patient guide is based on the NCCN Clinical Practice Guidelines in Oncology (NCCN Guidelines®) for Hodgkin Lymphoma, Version 2.2023. It was adapted, reviewed, and published with help from the following people:

Dorothy A. Shead, MS
Senior Director
Patient Information Operations

Erin Vidic, MA
Senior Medical Writer, Patient Information

Susan Kidney
Senior Graphic Design Specialist

The NCCN Clinical Practice Guidelines in Oncology (NCCN Guidelines®) for Hodgkin Lymphoma, Version 2.2023 were developed by the following NCCN Panel Members:

Richard T. Hoppe, MD/Chair
Stanford Cancer Institute

Ranjana H. Advani, MD/Vice Chair
Stanford Cancer Institute

Richard F. Ambinder, MD, PhD
The Sidney Kimmel Comprehensive Cancer Center at John Hopkins

Philippe Armand, MD, PhD
Dana-Farber/Brigham and Women's Cancer Center

*Celeste M. Bello, MD, MSPH
Moffitt Cancer Center

*Cecil M. Benitez, MD, PhD
UCLA Jonsson Comprehensive Cancer Center

Weina Chen, MD, PhD
UT Southwestern Simmons Comprehensive Cancer Center

Sheen Cherian, MD
Case Comprehensive Cancer Center/ University Hospitals Seidman Cancer Center and Cleveland Clinic Taussig Cancer Institute

Bouthaina Dabaja, MD
The University of Texas MD Anderson Cancer Center

Megan E. Daly, MD
UC Davis Comprehensive Cancer Center

Jamie Flerlage, MD, MS
St. Jude Children's Research Hospital/ The University of Tennessee Health Science Center

Leo I. Gordon, MD
Robert H. Lurie Comprehensive Cancer Center of Northwestern University

*Neil Hansen, MD
Fred & Pamela Buffett Cancer Center

Alex F. Herrera, MD
City of Hope National Medical Center

Ephraim P. Hochberg, MD
Massachusetts General Hospital Cancer Center

Patrick B. Johnston, MD, PhD
Mayo Clinic Cancer Center

Mark S. Kaminski, MD
University of Michigan Rogel Cancer Center

Christopher R. Kelsey, MD
Duke Cancer Institute

Vaishalee P. Kenkre, MD
University of Wisconsin Carbone Cancer Center

Ryan C. Lynch, MD
Fred Hutchinson Cancer Center

Kami Maddocks, MD
The Ohio State University Comprehensive Cancer Center- James Cancer Hospital and Solove Research Institute

Jonathan McConathy, MD, PhD
O'Neal Comprehensive Cancer Center at UAB

David Morgan, MD
Vanderbilt-Ingram Cancer Center

Carolyn Mulroney, MD
UC San Diego Moores Cancer Center

Sheeja T. Pullarkat, MD
UCLA Jonsson Comprehensive Cancer Center

Rachel Rabinovitch, MD
University of Colorado Cancer Center

Karen C. Rosenspire, MD, PhD
Abramson Cancer Center at the University of Pennsylvania

Stuart Seropian, MD
Yale Cancer Center/Smilow Cancer Hospital

*Michael Spinner, MD
UCSF Helen Diller Family Comprehensive Cancer Center

Randa Tao, MD
Huntsman Cancer Institute at the University of Utah

*Pallawi Torka, MD
Roswell Park Comprehensive Cancer Center

Jane N. Winter, MD
Robert H. Lurie Comprehensive Cancer Center of Northwestern University

Joachim Yahalom, MD
Memorial Sloan Kettering Cancer Center

Joanna C. Yang, MD, MPH
Siteman Cancer Center at Barnes-Jewish Hospital and Washington University School of Medicine

NCCN

Megan Lyons, MS
Guidelines Layout Specialist

Katie Stehman, PA-C, MMS
Oncology Scientist/Medical Writer

Hema Sundar, PhD
Manager, Global Clinical Content

* Reviewed this patient guide. For disclosures, visit NCCN.org/disclosures.

NCCN Cancer Centers

Abramson Cancer Center
at the University of Pennsylvania
Philadelphia, Pennsylvania
800.789.7366 • pennmedicine.org/cancer

Case Comprehensive Cancer Center/
University Hospitals Seidman Cancer
Center and Cleveland Clinic Taussig
Cancer Institute
Cleveland, Ohio
800.641.2422 • UH Seidman Cancer Center
uhhospitals.org/services/cancer-services
866.223.8100 • CC Taussig Cancer Institute
my.clevelandclinic.org/departments/cancer
216.844.8797 • Case CCC
case.edu/cancer

City of Hope National Medical Center
Duarte, California
800.826.4673 • cityofhope.org

Dana-Farber/Brigham and Women's
Cancer Center | Massachusetts
General Hospital Cancer Center
Boston, Massachusetts
617.732.5500 • youhaveus.org
617.726.5130
massgeneral.org/cancer-center

Duke Cancer Institute
Durham, North Carolina
888.275.3853 • dukecancerinstitute.org

Fox Chase Cancer Center
Philadelphia, Pennsylvania
888.369.2427 • foxchase.org

Fred & Pamela Buffett Cancer Center
Omaha, Nebraska
402.559.5600 • unmc.edu/cancercenter

Fred Hutchinson Cancer Center
Seattle, Washington
206.667.5000 • fredhutch.org

Huntsman Cancer Institute
at the University of Utah
Salt Lake City, Utah
800.824.2073 • huntsmancancer.org

Indiana University
Melvin and Bren Simon
Comprehensive Cancer Center
Indianapolis, Indiana
888.600.4822 • www.cancer.iu.edu

Mayo Clinic Cancer Center
Phoenix/Scottsdale, Arizona
Jacksonville, Florida
Rochester, Minnesota
480.301.8000 • Arizona
904.953.0853 • Florida
507.538.3270 • Minnesota
mayoclinic.org/cancercenter

Memorial Sloan Kettering
Cancer Center
New York, New York
800.525.2225 • mskcc.org

Moffitt Cancer Center
Tampa, Florida
888.663.3488 • moffitt.org

O'Neal Comprehensive
Cancer Center at UAB
Birmingham, Alabama
800.822.0933 • uab.edu/onealcancercenter

Robert H. Lurie Comprehensive Cancer
Center of Northwestern University
Chicago, Illinois
866.587.4322 • cancer.northwestern.edu

Roswell Park Comprehensive
Cancer Center
Buffalo, New York
877.275.7724 • roswellpark.org

Siteman Cancer Center at Barnes-
Jewish Hospital and Washington
University School of Medicine
St. Louis, Missouri
800.600.3606 • siteman.wustl.edu

St. Jude Children's
Research Hospital/
The University of Tennessee
Health Science Center
Memphis, Tennessee
866.278.5833 • stjude.org
901.448.5500 • uthsc.edu

Stanford Cancer Institute
Stanford, California
877.668.7535 • cancer.stanford.edu

The Ohio State University
Comprehensive Cancer Center -
James Cancer Hospital and
Solove Research Institute
Columbus, Ohio
800.293.5066 • cancer.osu.edu

The Sidney Kimmel Comprehensive
Cancer Center at Johns Hopkins
Baltimore, Maryland
410.955.8964
www.hopkinskimmelcancercenter.org

The University of Texas
MD Anderson Cancer Center
Houston, Texas
844.269.5922 • mdanderson.org

UC Davis
Comprehensive Cancer Center
Sacramento, California
916.734.5959 • 800.770.9261
health.ucdavis.edu/cancer

UC San Diego Moores Cancer Center
La Jolla, California
858.822.6100 • cancer.ucsd.edu

UCLA Jonsson
Comprehensive Cancer Center
Los Angeles, California
310.825.5268 • cancer.ucla.edu

UCSF Helen Diller Family
Comprehensive Cancer Center
San Francisco, California
800.689.8273 • cancer.ucsf.edu

University of Colorado Cancer Center
Aurora, Colorado
720.848.0300 • coloradocancercenter.org

University of Michigan
Rogel Cancer Center
Ann Arbor, Michigan
800.865.1125 • rogelcancercenter.org

University of Wisconsin
Carbone Cancer Center
Madison, Wisconsin
608.265.1700 • uwhealth.org/cancer

UT Southwestern Simmons
Comprehensive Cancer Center
Dallas, Texas
214.648.3111 • utsouthwestern.edu/simmons

Vanderbilt-Ingram Cancer Center
Nashville, Tennessee
877.936.8422 • vicc.org

Yale Cancer Center/
Smilow Cancer Hospital
New Haven, Connecticut
855.4.SMILOW • yalecancercenter.org

Index

Made in the USA
Monee, IL
05 November 2026

67379934R00040